Medical Intelligence Unit

Purging in Bone Marrow Transplantation

Subhash C. Gulati, M.D., Ph.D.

Memorial Sloan-Kettering Cancer Center
New York

R.G. Landes Company
Austin

MEDICAL INTELLIGENCE UNIT

PURGING IN BONE MARROW TRANSPLANTATION

R.G. LANDES COMPANY
Austin / Georgetown

CRC Press is the exclusive worldwide distributor of publications of the Medical Intelligence Unit.
CRC Press, 2000 Corporate Blvd., NW, Boca Raton, FL 33431. Phone: 407/994-0555.

Submitted: February 1993 / Published: April 1993
Second Printing: June 1993
Third Printing: October 1993

Production Manager: Terry Nelson
Copy Editor: Constance Kerkaporta

Please address all inquiries to the Publisher:
R.G. Landes Company, 909 Pine Street, Georgetown, TX 78626
or
P.O. Box 4858, Austin, TX 78765
Phone: 512/ 863 7762; FAX: 512/ 863 0081

ISBN 1-879702-56-8   CATALOG # LN0256

Library of Congress Cataloging-in-Publication
Gulati, Subhash C. (Subhash Chander, 1950-
Purging in bone marrow transplantation / Subhash C. Gulati.
p. cm. — (Medical intelligence unit)
Includes bibliographical references and index.
ISBN 1-879702-56-8: $89.95
1. Bone marrow purging. 2. Hematopoietic stem cells—Transplantation. I. Title. II. Series.
[DNLM: 1. Bone Marrow Purging. 2. Bone Marrow Transplantation—methods.
WH 380 G971p 1993]
RD123.5.G85 1993
617.4'4—dc20

DNLM/DLC
for Library of Congress

93-15292
CIP

CONTENTS

Dedication

To my parents and uncle Dr. Joginder Nath for their guidance, devotion and insights.

To my wife Cathy and my children Angeli, Tony and Nick for support and peace of mind to enable me to focus on my work.

To my teachers, co-workers and patients; without them this book would not be possible.

Acknowledgment

The generous support of the Tow Foundation, Lisa Bilotti Fund, The Lymphoma Foundation, Lauri Strauss Leukemia Foundation and Morgan Murray Fund and many other groups is greatly appreciated.

PREFACE

The use of bone marrow transplantation to reconstitute the hematopoietic system has been one of the major advances in medicine during the past few decades. Investigation in this area has stimulated the intensive study of transplantation biology, stem cell physiology, cryopreservation technology, selective cytotoxic agents, intensified systemic cancer therapy, immunological mechanisms, and detection of small numbers of genetically different cells.

In this monograph Dr. Subhash Gulati draws upon his extensive experience as head of the autologous bone marrow transplantation team and director of the bone marrow cryopreservation laboratory at Memorial Sloan-Kettering Cancer Center to deal with many of these areas. He describes in detail current approaches to processing and modifying harvested bone marrow, in order to optimize the chances for a successful clinical outcome.

In addition to reviewing procedures for eliminating undesired cells ("purging"), Dr. Gulati surveys current literature on efficacy of autologous bone marrow transplantation and outlines the many questions that still need to be addressed. He also discusses purging of immune cells from bone marrow that is being prepared for allogeneic transplantation. He presents the results of hematopoietic reconstruction studies substituting peripheral blood stem cells for bone marrow, and reviews the use of hematopoietic growth factors to enhance bone marrow recovery.

Dr. Gulati concludes that purging of bone marrow to remove malignant cells is already a promising approach in intensive therapy of the hematologic malignancies with autologous bone marrow rescue. However, he stresses the need for further investigation in the use of marrow rescue with both hematologic and solid tumors. His discussions of the unsolved problems in this field make it clear that a great deal of research remains to be done, especially at a time when costs of expensive medical therapies are being carefully weighed against objective data on benefits.

John Mendelsohn, M.D.
Chairman, Department of Medicine
Winthrop Rockefeller Chair in Medical Oncology
Memorial Sloan-Kettering Cancer Center

CHAPTER 1

HISTORY AND RATIONALE FOR PURGING

The success of cancer chemotherapy has improved markedly over the last 15 years. Greater than 50% of cancer patients can now have durable long-term disease free survival (LT-DFS).[1-6] The main reason for such success is better utilization of modern cytotoxic therapy. Also, improvements in supportive care for high dose chemotherapy have played an important role in increasing the survival of patients with many neoplastic diseases.[1-10] Higher dosages of chemotherapy are now being used with an intent of cure for many malignancies. The most common cytotoxic effect of such therapy is partial or complete ablation of the hematopoietic system. For that reason, over the last 15 years, various methods of hematopoietic support using either autologous bone marrow (AUBMT) or allogeneic bone marrow transplantation (ALBMT, especially when the patient's HLA compatible brother or sister is available) have been utilized. Recently, there has also been an increased use of hematopoietic growth factors (GM-CSF, G-CSF), and stem cells obtained from the patient's peripheral blood.[10-13] Furthermore, partially matched brother, sister or unrelated HLA matched donor transplantation[14,15] have also been utilized with improvement in hematopoietic reconstitution (Table 1). Various types of hematopoietic stem cell transplants are briefly detailed below:

1. In an *allogeneic bone marrow transplantation*, the patient's histocompatibility is determined with brothers and sisters. Usually one-third of the patients have an HLA compatible sibling. Partially matched family member transplants have also been performed with reasonable success especially in younger patients.[7,8,16,17]

2. *Autologous bone marrow transplantation* (AUBMT) involves the use of the patient's own bone marrow. For technical reasons, the optimum time for freezing such cells is very important for the overall success of high dose chemotherapy followed by AUBMT. The bone marrow may be contaminated with cancer cells and it is important to develop methods for selective elimination (purging) of the cancer cells from the bone marrow. Various approaches are available for such purging.[3,9,18-21]

3. In the past years (Table 2), there has been an increased use of the patient's *peripheral blood stem cells* (PBSC) transplantation. These cells can be obtained in higher quantities if they are primed by prior chemotherapy or by the use of hematopoietic growth factors. There is a suggestion that platelet

Table 1. Methods of hematopoietic reconstitution

Type of Transplant	Major Advantages	Major Disadvantages
ALLOGENEIC		
HLA-MLC compatible family member	Good engraftment	Compatible donor available 30%-35%
	Graft vs cancer effect	Graft vs host disease
		Interstitial pneumonia
		Cytomegaloviral infection
		Increased risks with age
HLA-MLC compatible unrelated donor	Engraftment	Graft rejection
(? cadaveric source)	Greater graft vs cancer effect	Purging lymphocytes can alter
or		engraftment
HLA-MLC partially matched family member		
HLA-MLC unrelated donor; 1 to 3 loci mismatch;		
Umbilical Blood		
(?Fetal hematopoietic cells)		
SYNGENEIC		
HLA-MLC compatible monozygotic twin	Excellent engraftment	Increased risk of relapse
AUTOLOGOUS		
Bone Marrow	Good engraftment	No graft vs cancer effect
Peripheral Blood Cells	No need to look for a donor	Risk of relapse from the infused
Cultured Cells	Success with older patients	hematopoietic stem cells
	Lower risk of Cytomegalovirus infection	Graft failure:
		1. Effect of previous Rx
		2. Purging conditions

Table 2. Development of PBSC transplantation technology

Cavin (1962): Lethally irradiated dogs can be rescued by PB.

Bradley & Metcalf (1966), McCredie (1971): PB contains CFU-GM.

Micklen (1975): PB failed in hematopoietic reconstitution of mice.

Riechman (1976): Chemotherapy increases PBSC in humans.

Barrett (1978): Exercise, ACTH, DEXTRAN increase PBSC number.

Kovacs (1978): Repeated leukopheresis increases PBSC in dogs.

Goldman (1979): PBSC used for transplantation in CML.

Abrams (1981): CTX expands PBSC.

To (1984): Increased PBSC in AML patients recovering.

Reiffers (1986): PBSC used for transplantation in AML.

Kessingers (1986): PBSC for transplantation in lymphoma.

Gianni (1988): Growth factor and/or CTX priming expands PBSC.

Source: Abstracted from [9, 10, 23]

count recovery is faster when PBSC are utilized. There is some evidence that peripheral blood stem cells contain less contamination by the cancer cells than the bone marrow.[22,23] Further experiments are needed to prove the therapeutic benefit of peripheral blood stem cells over AUBMT especially in heavily pretreated patients. Purging of PBSC is usually not performed, but can be considered in the future.

4. *Matched unrelated donors.* In the past 10 years, there has been a unified effort in finding HLA/MLC compatible donors for "matched unrelated bone marrow transplantation". Such transplantations have been successful when a suitable HLA/MLC compatible donor is available, especially for young patients. National registries are now helping patients find such unrelated donors. There is, however, a significant complication of graft-versus-host disease even though various methods of depleting T-lymphocytes from such donor harvest have been very useful in improving the quality of the hematopoietic engraftment.[14-17] Further investigations are needed to make this technique widely applicable for patient use as the relapse rate may increase following T-lymphocyte depletion.[24,25] In addition, some investigators are evaluating the feasibility of cadaveric bone marrow transplantation.

5. *Umbilical blood.* It has been known for a long time that mononuclear cells obtained from the umbilical blood are able to adopt to a new host without any significant problem of graft rejection or graft-versus-host disease. Umbilical blood, especially when cells expanded with the use of hematopoietic growth factors are used, should be able to reconstitute the hematopoietic system. The early data appear very promising.[26-28]

6. *Splenic and other cells.* In animal model systems, splenic and liver cells are a rich source of hematopoietic cells and transplants using human fetal tissue have been successful in hematopoietic reconstitution.[29-30]

The risk of concomitant cancer cell infusion with hematopoietic stem cell support in autologous stem cell transplant (utilizing bone marrow or PBSC,

AUSCT) or complications of graft-versus-host disease from the infused cells in allogeneic bone marrow transplant has been known for a long time. For this reason, various methods to eliminate "the problem cell" by purging methods have been attempted for many years. Diseases which may benefit from purged BMT are listed in Table 3. The complications caused by infused cancer cells in AUSCT or by lymphocytes in ALBMT will be diminished if

---

Table 3. Partial list of diseases which may benefit from purged BMT

MALIGNANT DISORDERS
Leukemias
    1. Acute lymphoblastic leukemia (ALL)
    2. Acute non-lymphoblastic leukemia (AML, ANNL)
    3. Chronic Myelogenous Leukemia (CML)
Lymphomas
    1. Hodgkin's
    2. Non-Hodgkin's
Multiple myeloma, CLL
Myelodysplastic syndrome
Solid tumors
    1. Brain tumors
    2. Breast cancer
    3. Germ cells tumors (testicular, extra-gonadal)
    4. Neuroblastoma
    5. Ovarian cancer
    6. Sarcomas (Ewing's, Rhabdomyosarcoma)

NON-MALIGNANT DISORDERS
Acquired
    1. Aplastic anemia
    2. Paroxysmal nocturnal hemoglobinuria
    3. Myelofibrosis
*Congenital
    1. Immunodeficiency Syndromes
        a. Severe combined immunodeficiency syndrome (SCID)
        b. Chronic mucocutaneous candidiasis
        c. Wiscott-Aldrich syndrome
    2. Hematologic Defects
        a. Hemoglobinopathies
          - Sickle cell anemia
          - Thalassemia
        b. Fanconi's anemia
        c. Diamond-Blackfan anemia
        d. Congenital neutropenia
        e. Chronic granulomatous disease
        f. Chediak-Hagashi syndrome
        g. Gaucher's disease
    3. Lysosomal diseases (Lesch-Nyhan syndrome)
    4. Mucolipidoses (Metachromatic leukodystrophy)
    5. Mucopolysaccharidoses (Hurler syndrome, Hunter syndrome)
    6. Osteopetrosis
* Enzyme replacement, gene therapy may also have clinical benefit.

the appropriate cells are preferentially reduced. In ALBMT, it may be preferable to use bone marrow (BM) over PBSC as the PBSC contain more lymphocytes. In AUSCT, quantity and quality of stem cells obtained vary depending on the patient's diagnosis, stage, therapy and treatment induced side effects. One of the initial trials for successfully eliminating cancer cells from the infused stem cells in a rat model was performed at Johns Hopkins.[31] A drug, 4-hydroperoxycyclophosphamide (4-HC) was developed; it is an active analog of cyclophosphamide and upon placing it in aqueous solution, it spontaneously converts itself into the biologically active phosphoramide mustard form. Cyclophosphamide, on the other hand, needs to be activated by liver microsomes. Sharkis et al[31] first demonstrated that 4-HC treatment of a bone marrow graft in vitro could eliminate tumor cells while sparing enough normal marrow cells to allow engraftment after bone marrow transplantation (BMT). A rat model of autologous BMT, which employed syngeneic BMT of bone marrow mixed with the transplantable rat acute myeloid leukemia cells, was used in this study. All rats transplanted with 64×10^6 marrow cells mixed with 1×10^6 leukemia cells died of leukemia, as did all mice transplanted with the same graft treated with 20 nmoles/ml 4-HC for 30 minutes at $37°C$. However, about one-third of rats transplanted with grafts purged with 40 nmoles/ml 4-HC and essentially all mice transplanted with grafts purged with 60-80 nmoles/ml 4-HC survived long-term. Further increases in the 4-HC concentration produced increasing death rates resulting from marrow aplasia.

Since these early experiments, 4-HC has been widely used for clinical trials involving purging. In the subsequent chapters, the results of 4-HC purged bone marrow transplantation will be reviewed.[9,18,19] Other analogs of cyclophosphamide have also given comparable results.[32] (See also Chapter 4.) In addition, monoclonal antibodies specific against various malignancies have been the subject of intense investigation for proper use in purging autologous bone marrow transplant.[18-21,33] Several centers have developed antibodies specific against lymphoma, leukemia, small cell lung cancer and neuroblastoma. These antibodies are in various stages of clinical investigations. The antibodies can be used to lyse the subject cells by complement, radioactivity or toxins; or used to separate the subject cell by immunomagnetic beads or avidin-biotin column separation. Antibodies are also available to deplete the lymphocytes prior to infusion of bone marrow for allogeneic BMT. This method decreases GVHD. Furthermore, toxin conjugated antibodies can treat GVHD once it has been established in the patients.[24,25,34] Specific purging methods are detailed in Chapter 2.

SIGNIFICANT ISSUES IN AUTOLOGOUS BONE MARROW TRANSPLANTATION

OPTIMUM TIMING OF STEM CELL HARVEST

Various factors must be considered in regard to timing of the stem cell harvest. The clinical situation for each disease (especially where bone marrow is involved) and its appropriate therapy have to be considered. These issues include: (1) How likely is it that a stem cell transplant will be needed? (2) Is the bone marrow involved? (3) Will therapy result in improvement of the bone marrow function? (4) Will it be better to harvest hematopoietic stem cells when the tumor burden is at the lowest level? (5) Should bone marrow and/or peripheral blood stem cells be harvested? (6) Will therapy result in transient or permanent damage to the hematopoietic stem cells? Unfortunately, it is very hard to design scientifically meaningful clinical trials to properly understand the importance of the issues discussed above.

Most investigators believe that busulfan, carmustine, and bleomycin are more damaging to stem cells, but the effect of quantity and duration of exposure in patients exposed to multiple drugs is not scientifically easy to evaluate. Interesting approaches to help predict stem cell toxicity have been developed. In an in vivo murine model,[35] effects of a number of individual cytotoxic agents on the ability of syngeneic donor marrow to provide long-term hematopoiesis in recipients following high-dose total body irradiation were evaluated. Marrow was obtained after giving donor mice six weekly injections of saline, cytosine arabinoside, cyclophosphamide, cisplatin, 1,3-bis(2-chloroethyl)-1-nitrosourea (BCNU), or busulfan (drugs known to have different effects on primitive hematopoietic stem cells). After allowing time for recovery of marrow and peripheral blood counts, 1×10^7 marrow cells from these mice were transplanted into lethally irradiated syngeneic recipients. Five to six months after marrow transplantation, the quality of long-term hematopoietic recovery was measured by WBC counts, marrow cellularity, CFU-S content, and determinations of stem cell self-renewal. Abnormalities were noted with the use of donor marrow exposed to all cytotoxic agents. Recipients of marrow previously exposed to cytosine arabinoside, an agent that spares the most primitive stem cells, were the least affected. Recipients of marrow previously exposed to busulfan, an agent known to damage primitive stem cells, were most affected with a decrease in peripheral blood counts, marrow cellularity, stem cell content, self-renewal capacity, and long-term survival. A decrease in hematopoietic stem cell self-renewal was seen in recipients of marrow previously exposed to cyclophosphamide, cisplatin, and BCNU even when marrow cellularity and CFU-S content were normal. These data suggest that the capacity of syngeneic donor marrow to provide long-term hematopoiesis in lethally irradiated recipients is dependent on its donor marrow "early progenitor stem cell" content. Long-term hematopoiesis may be severely compromised in recipients of donor stem cells previously exposed to cytotoxic agents which damage primitive stem cells.[35] One recommendation is that patients who are eligible for stem cell harvesting (bone marrow or peripheral blood), should not have recent exposure to stem cell-damaging agents, and if exposed, the blood counts should be in the recovery phase. Preferably, the leukocyte count should be greater than 3000/mm³ and platelets greater than 100,000/mm³.

ROLE OF DISEASE ERADICATION IN VIVO VERSUS EX VIVO

Even with the advent of improved technologies, our ability to detect small amounts of cancer cells contaminating the stem cell harvest is poor.[18-22] Specific antibodies can detect perhaps one in a million cells for neuroblastoma, small cell lung cancer and other similar cancers. Flow cytometric analysis helps detect a rare aneuploid cancer cell. Polymerase chain reaction is not applicable in most clinical situations, as it is often too sensitive, and has frequent laboratory errors. Recent use of fluorescence in situ hybridization

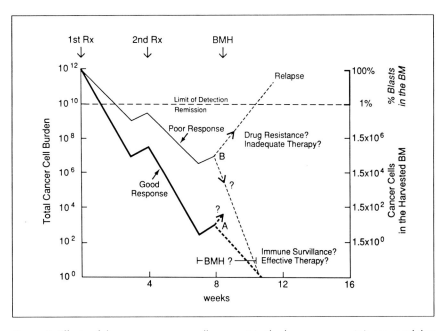

Figure 1. Effects of therapy on cancer cells present in the bone marrow. It is assumed that one kilogram of cancer would fully replace bone marrow (100% blasts in case of leukemia). With effective therapy, three to five log reduction is expected. The model assumes regrowth of disease during the recovery phase after each therapy. Most patients will have undetectable disease below the dotted line but variable amounts of cancer cells will still be harvested in situation A versus situation B. Assuming patients weight to be 75 kilogram and 200 million cells per kilogram patients weight are harvested, the cancer cells present in the bone marrow harvest are estimated on the right side of the graph.

technology or careful use of polymerase chain reaction may be useful in the future. (See also Chapter 6.) Figure 1 describes the number of cancer cells that still might persist after using the best therapy for acute leukemia. When the best diagnostic tools fail to reveal involvement of the bone marrow, minimal contamination with cancer cell may still be present. Purging of stem cells in such conditions with minimal disease will most likely be better than ex vivo manipulation when a greater number of cancer cells are present. Thus, we favor the concept that ex vivo (purging) treatment will be most useful in patients with minimal disease at stem cell harvest.

Recurrence from Persistent Disease Versus Infused Stem Cell Contamination

In patients who relapse after autologous stem cell transplantation (AUSCT), it is often impossible to predict if the recurrence occurred from the infused cells or from inadequate treatment of the patient. Perhaps recurrence in the liver, lung (sites where infused stem cells transiently persist prior to homing in the bone marrow), and bone marrow may suggest relapse from infused stem cell contamination. In the future, genetic engineering may provide markers to help track the in vitro manipulated and subsequently transplanted cells.[36] In a recent study,[21] clonogenic assays were performed using a tumor cell line in culture to determine the efficiency of immunologic purging. Amplification by polymerase chain reaction was subsequently used to detect residual lymphoma cells "before and after" purging of bone marrow from 114 patients with B-cell, non-Hodgkin's lymphoma in whom a translocation [t(14;18)] with presence of bcl-2 gene that could be amplified by polymerase chain reaction] was detected at the time of initial evaluation. Immunologic purging in vitro resulted in a 3- to 6-log destruction of cells in the tumor cell line. Residual lymphoma cells were detected by polymerase chain reaction in the bone marrow of all patients before purging. No lymphoma cells could be detected in the marrow of 57 patients after purging. Disease-free survival was increased in these 57 patients as compared to those whose marrow contained detectable residual lymphoma (p<0.00001). The ability to purge residual lymphoma cells was not associated with the degree of bone marrow involvement (P=0.4994) or the previous response to therapy (P=0.1298). The ability to purge residual lymphoma cells was the most important prognostic indicator in predicting relapse.[21] These results provide evidence of the clinical usefulness of ex vivo purging of autologous bone marrow in the treatment of patients with lymphoma and suggest that the reinfusion of malignant cells in autologous marrow contributes to relapse. Further studies are needed to confirm this observation and to use these methods for other diseases and purging techniques.

The Need For Hematopoietic Rescue In Autologous Bone Marrow Transplantation

Various approaches can be used for hematopoietic rescue. In trials reporting hematopoietic recovery soon after the completion of cytotoxic therapy, the need for the stem cell rescue can be questioned. Table 4 describes the single drug dosage which usually requires stem cell support.[9,37] Avoiding stem

Table 4. Effect of single agent dose (mg/m²) and need for hematopoietic stem cell (HSC) rescue

Drug	Usual Maximum Dose Without HSC Rescue Often with G-CSF or GM-CSF	Usual Maximum Dose with HSC Rescue	Non-Hematopoietic Toxicity
BCNU	100 - 200	300 - 900	Pulmonary, Hepatic
Busulfan	4 - 6	600	Hepatic, Pulmonary
Carboplatin	400 - 1,200	2,000 - 2,400	Hepatic
Cisplatin	100 - 120	150 - 200	Renal
Cyclophosphamide	3,000	6,000 - 7,500	Cardiac, GU
Etoposide	800 - 1,200	1,800 - 2,400	GI
Ifosfamide	5,000 - 8,000	12,000 - 16,000	CNS, GU
Melphalan	30	100 - 200	GI
Mitomycin-C	10	40 - 60	Cardiac, Hepatic, Pulmonary
Mitoxantrone	30	60	GI, Hepatic
TBI	100 Rads	1,300 - 1,500	Hepatic, Pulmonary
Thiotepa	120	750 - 1,200	CNS, GI

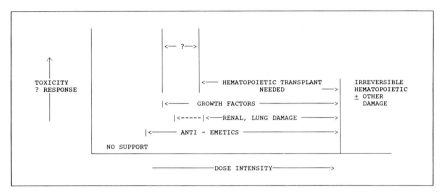

Figure 2. Supportive care depends on the drug dose. Need for various support methods is different for each cytotoxic agent. Growth factors may stimulate recovery of hematopoietic cells (GM-CSF, G-CSF, erythropoietin, etc.) or may protect normal cells from the injury of the cytotoxic drugs (TGF-ß, MIF, etc).

cell rescue in such situations will decrease the complications associated with stem cell transplantation. Furthermore, one can explore dose escalation with the use of hematopoietic growth factors (without stem cell transplantation). In this regard, there is also an interest in giving conventional or intermediate drug dose over shorter periods of time to evaluate the benefit of dose intensity. Figure 2 describes the need to properly understand the maximum drug dosage which can be safely administered without the need of hematopoietic support. In animal studies, syngeneic chromosomal markers prove that hematopoietic recovery is from the transplanted cells. However, in human AUSCT trials, it is more difficult to prove that the transplanted stem cells are responsible for engraftment. If previous experience with ALBMT has already proven the hematoablative potential of treatment, then it is usually safe to assume that the same high-dose therapy in AUSCT will need stem cell rescue. The role of stem cell rescue for newer drug combinations can be evaluated by the following approaches.[18]

One method would be to perform dose escalation studies with stem cells available as back-up. In this situation, the stem cells are infused only if the hematopoietic recovery has not taken place after approximately 15 to 28 days. Unfortunately, the hematopoietic engraftment in different patients is variable and scientific proof may be hard to establish. The morbidity and mortality will be high and the risk of disease recurrence by infused bone marrow will be low. Another approach is to conduct dose escalation studies and rescue all patients with stem cells. Under such conditions, nonhematologic, i.e., heart, lung, kidney, toxicity will be dose limiting and the therapeutic benefits of each dose level can be properly evaluated. If at the highest useful drug dose level, the hematopoietic engraftment is too fast (within 10 to 15 days), then 5 to 10 patients can be considered for treatment at that dose level without upfront stem cell rescue to prove the need for transplant. A third approach would be to conduct the above studies with growth factor support alone or in combination with HSC rescue.

How many patients can be entered onto each part of the study will depend on the goals of the investigator (Table 5). Most publications detail tolerability, studies should be designed to specifically prove the usefulness of

Table 5. Approaches to dose escalation studies

A. 1. Tolerability: First Study (4-10 patients)
    2. Clinical Benefit: Second Study (10 or more patients)
    3. Phase III comparison

B. Tolerability and clinical benefit simultaneously (usually 15-30 patients) for drugs with reasonable track record (CTX, VP-16, Carboplatinum, etc). This approach will avoid unnecessary dose escalation and may not require hematopoietic stem cell rescue.

Table 6. Major issues regarding purging for transplantation

Proof that high dose cytotoxic therapy was needed (when, how frequently)?

Proof that BMT or PBSCT was needed?

Can hematopoeitic growth factors eliminate the need of transplant?

How many cells are needed for hematopoietic engraftment?

Does inadvertent infusion of cancer cells with stem cells (BM and/or PB) increase relapse?

Does purging work ex-vivo?

Does purging have clinical benefit?

How to quantitate minimal disease and it's impact on clinical course?

Do processing methods injure stem cells?

Role and side effects of supportive therapy (GM-CSF, G-CSF, etc.)?

Role of post-transplant therapy?

For allogeneic BMT: Graft-versus-cancer effect?

Quality of life after various types of transplant?

Clinical and cost benefit?

each step as the current data does not strongly prove the clinical benefit of the multiple manipulations performed for autologous stem cell transplant (Table 6). Increased dose intensity is usually associated with lower relapse rate for patients with Hodgkin's disease, lymphoma, breast cancer, etc., but there are also situations where the increased drug dose has not correlated with decrease in relapse rate. Therefore, each disease will have a different "drug-dose escalation versus response" curve (Figure 2).[1,9,38-40]

SIGNIFICANT ISSUES RELATED TO ALLOGENEIC BONE MARROW TRANSPLANTATION

In patients undergoing ALBMT, the cytotoxic conditioning regimen must ablate the host immune system along with the hematopoietic compartment. That donor cells have reconstituted the hematopoietic system is easy to prove by appropriate studies (see below). Often, a mixed chimeric state persists.[14-17,41-56] Patients are monitored for changes in hematopoietic reconstitution and for the development of graft-versus-host disease (GVHD). Occurrence of GVHD and graft failure depends on several factors. The most important is thought to be the number of T-cells present in the infused BM, other factors include conditioning regimen (especially the mode of TBI), prophylactic therapy, etc.[44-50] Patients receiving T lymphocyte-depleted bone marrow transplantation often experience a higher incidence of graft rejection. Several approaches are being investigated to optimize the bone marrow purging conditions. These techniques are also useful when unrelated donors are considered for transplantation. Commonly used methods for T lymphocyte depletion include: 1.Soybean agglutinin (lectin) bind to specific membrane receptors; and T lymphocytes can be selectively removed by agglutination. This technique is usually combined with sheep erythrocytes rosetting to further purge the T lymphocytes.[24,25] 2. Antibodies to selectively eliminate all T-lymphocytes or its subsets.[46-50]

In one recent study,[14] 112 patients less than 36 years old, received marrow grafts from unrelated donors as treatment for hematologic malignancy. Seventy donor/recipient pairs were phenotypically identical for HLA-A, -B, and -D, while 42 had a "minor" disparity at one HLA locus. There was an increase in the risk of acute graft-versus-host disease (GVHD) in patients receiving HLA-partially matched grafts compared to those receiving HLA-matched grafts (51% v 36% probability of grades III-IV acute GVHD). However, in this cohort of patients, there was no significant difference in survival (at 1.5 years, 46% v 51% for good-risk patients, 44% v 30% for poor-risk patients). This finding suggests that some degree of HLA disparity can be tolerated in young patients transplanted from unrelated donors for malignant disease.

Several techniques have been used to evaluate how the infused donor marrow is engrafting in relation to host hematopoietic cells. Transient presence of both host and donor cells (chimerism) in the hematopoietic system after allogeneic BMT is well-known. Methods used to detect mixed chimerism have included red blood cell (RBC) polymorphisms, cytogenetic analysis and fluorescent in situ hybridization. These techniques can be unreliable due to limited degree of polymorphism, poor sensitivity, RBC transfusions or the requirement for a donor and recipient that are sex-mismatched. More recently, chimerism has been evaluated using DNA restriction fragment length polymorphisms (RFLP), which are created by either the loss or gain of a restriction enzyme cleavage site or by the insertion or deletion of DNA between restriction sites. Determining both myeloid and lymphoid chimerism after T-cell-depleted allogeneic bone marrow transplantation (BMT) could be helpful in the understanding of the biology of engraftment and could provide a rational method of assessing the ability of different conditioning regimens to promote engraftment.

Mackinnon et al prospectively investigated the role of different pretransplant conditioning regimens of 29 leukemic patients post-BMT by assessing myeloid and T-cell chimerism using a rapid and sensitive polymerase chain reaction (PCR) method.[44] In each cell, mini-satellites were present and were derived from hypervariable regions of DNA consisting of tandem repeats of a core nucleotide sequence and allelic polymorphism resulting from differences in the number of the repeats. This variation was used to distinguish between donor and recipient cells post-BMT. Seventeen patients (9 sibling and 8 unrelated donors) received conditioning with hyperfractionated total body irradiation (TBI), thiotepa, and cyclophospha-mide (Cy). Of the other 12 patients (all sibling donors), 11 received TBI plus Cy plus another agent: VP-16, carboplatinum, or AZQ. One patient received TBI plus thiotepa plus VP-16. All but one of the patients studied received marrow from HLA-identical donors. PCR analysis confirmed donor lym-phoid engraftment within 8 days of transplant in six of six patients studied. All granulocyte DNA was of donor origin within the first 4 weeks of trans-plant, regardless of the conditioning regimen. The day +28 T-cells were exclusively of donor origin in 14 of 17 patients who received TBI plus thiotepa plus Cy, but were mixed chimeric in 10 of 12 patients who received other conditioning regimens (P<.001). Early graft rejection was seen in one unrelated transplant recipient conditioned with TBI plus thiotepa plus Cy. Late graft failure was observed in 3 of 12 patients with mixed T-cell chimer-ism and in none of 16 patients with full donor chimerism at day +28. However, 5 of 16 patients who had complete T-cell chimerism at day +28 developed acute graft-versus-host disease (GVHD), whereas no patient with mixed chimerism had acute GVHD. The results indicate that mini-satellite PCR is a rapid and sensitive method for assessing chimerism post-BMT, that the donor T-cells are important for consistent durable engraftment, and that TBI plus thiotepa plus Cy may be superior to the other regimens studied in inducing full donor chimerism.[44] Larger number of patients and longer follow-up are necessary to confirm these data and also to assess the relation-ship between complete donor T-cell chimerism and leukemia-free survival.

GRAFT-VERSUS-CANCER EFFECT

Investigators have noted a higher relapse rate when a syngeneic sibling is used for transplantation. Furthermore, patients developing mild GVHD tend to have better survival than patients with severe GVHD. Modulation of GVHD (by T-cell add back, IL-2 therapy, cyclosporine) might be useful;[51-57] several investigators are exploring its role in decreasing relapse. Our under-standing of graft-versus-host disease has improved.[55] It was initially thought that acute GVHD was caused by T-lymphocytes contained in the donor graft that recognized antigenic disparities between donor and recipient. Efforts to control GVHD were therefore directed against the donor-derived T-cell. For example, prophylactic use of cyclosporine ameliorated GVHD most likely by inhibiting the increased expression of interleukin-2 (IL-2) and IL-2 receptors (IL-2R) by T-lymphocytes during T-cell activation. Methotrexate is cytotoxic towards T-lymphocytes that are proliferating in response to stimulation by recipient antigens. Depleting the graft of T-cells by a variety of techniques can reduce GVHD by limiting the number of alloreactive cells in the infused marrow. However, both pharmacologic prophylaxis of GVHD and T-cell deple-tion have substantial pitfalls. Cyclosporine, methotrexate, corticosteroids, and other drugs are not completely effective in controlling GVHD.[53,55] Furthermore, the patient is subject to significant drug-related toxicity. T-cell depletion is more effective than pharmacologic prophylaxis at preventing GVHD, but is associated with a higher risk of graft rejection as well as loss of the graft-versus-leukemia

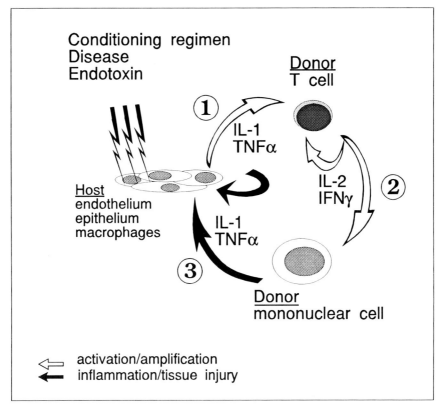

Figure 3. Schematic representation of the role of inflammatory cytokines in acute GVHD. In step 1, injury to host tissues, either directly by the conditioning regimen or indirectly through the production of cytokines, results in alterations in the host tissues, such as increased expression of HLA molecules, adhesion molecules, procoagulants, etc. In step 2, mature T-cells infused with the bone marrow respond to these changes in the allogeneic host tissues. This response includes the autocrine production of IL-2 and IFN-γ, which in turn activate mononuclear cell effectors from donor marrow. In step 3, additional production of inflammatory cytokines by these donor mononuclear cells results in direct tissue injury. Endotoxin released by gram-negative bacteria as well as production of other cytokines such as IL-6, IL-8, and NKSF may further amplify the injury and recruit additional effectors. Reproduced with permission from Blood.[55]

(GVL) effect, an important adjunct in the control of leukemia.[55]

An ideal prophylactic regimen would reduce the organ damage associated with GVHD and would not impair hematopoietic engraftment and the graft-versus-cancer (GVC) effect. It is likely that the development of such a regimen will require new insights into the pathophysiology of GVHD. Recent data suggest that mechanisms other than direct T-cell-mediated cytotoxicity may generate tissue damage associated with GVHD. Indeed, several convergent lines of evidence implicate a network of inflammatory cytokines as primary mediators of acute GVHD (Figure 3).[55] One suggestion is that acute GVHD after marrow transplantation reflects (1) host injury due to the conditioning regimen followed by the production of inflammatory cytokines; (2) stimulation of mature donor T-cells in the milieu of increased cell surface expression of leukocyte adhesion molecules and HLA molecules, followed by the autocrine production of IL-2; and finally, (3) recruitment and activation of additional mononuclear effector cells from donor marrow progenitors, which produce additional inflammatory cytokines, thus sustaining the response. The second step is critical for the amplification of the systemic inflammatory response, and it is probably absent in autologous, syngeneic and T cell-depleted transplants. These T-cells may also contribute to the inflammatory cytokine network. Acute GVHD can occur in the absence of primary tissue injury in such settings as transfusion-related GVHD; however, it is likely that a greater HLA disparity between donor and host is required. It is proposed that inflammatory cytokine production is the final common pathway of acute GVHD.[55] If this model is correct, control of cytokine disregulation at any of several points should control GVHD. Further studies of GVHD and investigations of cytokine antagonists, e.g., IL-4 or IL-10, or combinations of antagonists such as IL-1 receptor antagonist and soluble TNF receptor or pentoxifylline will allow us to determine the validity of this hypothesis.[55,56] Transient GVHD can be caused with proper use of cyclosporine or by infusing small amounts of mononuclear cells or purified lymphocytes. Such approaches should only be used with careful planning and as part of clinical research trials. Recent evidence suggests that the immunoregulatory mechanisms may also play a crucial role in the clearance of minimal cancer burden. Patients with low interleukin-2-mediated lymphocyte activated killer cell activity are expected to have a higher risk of relapse. The role of immunomodulation in this regard is being further explored.[55,58]

In patients undergoing ALBMT, recurrence of cancer cells (especially in leukemia patients) is usually of host origin, but leukemia in the donor cells has been occasionally described. We still need to understand more about the biology of leukemia and complex changes which occur with ALBMT. Frequently, patients undergoing cardiac, renal and bone marrow transplantation develop lymphoma, probably due to immunosuppression. These lymphomas are most often associated with Epstein-Barr virus. The role of EBV in this situation needs further investigations. Novel therapies for these lymphomas have recently been described.[59] The ultimate success of patients undergoing transplantation will not only depend on the most efficient hematopoietic rescue but also on the optimum use of the best conditioning regimen used for in vivo eradication of the disease. Optimum timing for such conditioning regimen will help lower the tumor burden and also decrease toxicity. Particular emphasis in this regard also needs to be placed on managing the non-hematopoietic toxicity of the transplant conditioning regimen.

It is better to know some of the questions than all of the answers.
                    —James Thurber (1894-1961)

From the issues discussed in this chapter and briefly detailed in Table 6, it is important that we properly prove the clinical benefit of each step as it relates to purging and subsequently to the success of BMT. Each investigator will have to decide which question is the most important to them. At this time, considerable conflicting results favor one approach over the other. The following chapters describe the present knowledge and also discuss strategies to prove the clinical benefit of purging.

REFERENCES

1. Devita VT, Hubbard SM, Longo DL: The chemotherapy of lymphoma; looking back, moving forward. The Richard and Hinda Rosenthal foundation award lecture. Cancer Research 1987; 47:5810-5824.
2. DeVita VT, Sepick AA, Carbone PP: Combination chemotherapy in the treatment of advanced Hodgkin's disease. Ann Intern Med 1970; 73:881-895.
3. Cheson DB, Leocadio L, Leyland-Jones J: Autologous bone marrow trans-plantation: current status and future directions. Ann Int Med 1989; 110:51-65.
4. Bonadonna G, Valagussa P, Santoro A: Alternating non-cross-resistant combination chemotherapy with ABVD or MOPP in Hodgkin's disease: a report of eight years results. Ann Intern Med 1986; 104:739-746.
5. Einhorn LH: Testicular cancer as a model for curable neoplasm. The Richard and Hinda Rosenthal Foundation Award Lecture. Cancer Research 1981; 41:3275-3280.
6. Frei E III, Kass F, Weeks J: Quality of life in cancer patients: clinical considerations and perspectives. Oncology 1990; 4:204-207.
7. Thomas ED: Marrow transplantation for malignant diseases: Karnofsky memorial lecture. J Clin Oncol 1983; 1:517-531.
8. O'Reilly, RJ: Allogeneic bone marrow transplantation: Current status and future directions. Blood 1983; 62:941-964.
9. Gulati SC, Yahalom J, Portlock C: Autologous bone marrow transplantation. Current problems in Cancer 1991; 15:1-57.
10. Gianni AM, Bregni M, Siena S, Orazi A, Stern AC, Gandola L, Bonadonna G: Recombinant human granulocyte-macrophage colony-stimulating factor reduces hematologic toxicity and widens clinical applicability of high-dose cyclophosphamide treatment in breast cancer and non-Hodgkin's lymphoma. Journal of Clinical Oncology 1990; 8:768-778.
11. Gabrilove JL, Jakubowski A, Scher H, Sternberg C, Wong G, Grous J, Yagoda A, Fain K, Moore MAS, Clarkson B, Oettgen HF, Alton K, Welte K, Souza L: Effect of granulocyte colony-stimulating factor on neutropenia and associated morbidity due to chemotherapy for transitional-cell carcinoma of the urothelium. New England Journal of Medicine 1988; 318:1414-1422.
12. Antman KS, Griffin JD, Elias A, Socinski MA, Ryan L, Cannistra SA, Oette D, Whitley M, Frei III E, Schnipper LE: Effect of recombinant human granulocyte-macrophage colony-stimulating factor on chemo-therapy-induced myelosuppression. New England Journal of Medicine 1988; 319:593-598.
13. Gulati SC, Bennett CL: Granulocyte-Macrophage Colony-Stimulating Factor (GM-CSF) as Adjunct Therapy in Relapsed Hodgkin's Disease. Ann Intern Med 1992; 116:177-182.
14. Beatty PG, Anasetti C, Hansen JA, Longton GM, Sanders JE, Martin PJ, Mickelson EM, Choo SY, Petersdorf EW, Pepe MS, Appelbaum FR, Bearman SI, Buckner CD, Clift RA, Petersen FB, Singer J, Stewart PS, Storb RF, Sullivan KM, Tesler MC, Witherspoon RP, Thomas ED: Marrow transplantation from unrelated donors for treatment of hemato-logic malignancies: Effect of mismatching for one HLA Locus. Blood

1993; 81:249-253.

15. McGlave PB, Beatty PG, Ash R, Hows JM: Therapy of chronic myelog-enous leukemia with unrelated donor bone marrow transplantation. Results in 102 cases. Blood 1990; 75:1728-1732.

16. Anasetti C, Beatty PG, Storb R, Martin PJ, Mori M, Sanders JE, Thomas ED, Hansen JA: Effect of HLA incompatibility on graft-versus-host disease, relapse, and survival after marrow transplantation for patients with leukemia or lymphoma, Human Immunol 1990; 29:79.

17. McGlave P, Bartsch G, Anasetti C, Ash R, Beatty P, Gajewski J, Kernan NA: Unrelated Donor Marrow Transplantation Therapy for Chronic Myelogenous Leukemia: Initial Experience of the National Marrow Donor Program. Blood 1993; 81:543-550.

18. Gulati SC, Lemoli RM, Acaba L, Igarashi T, Wasserheit C, Fraig M: Purging in autologous and allogeneic bone marrow transplantation. Current Opinion in Onc 1992; 4:264-271.

19. Shpall EJ, Johnson C, Hami L: Bone marrow purging, In: Armitage JO and Antman KH, ed. High dose cancer therapy. Baltimore, Maryland: Williams and Wilkins Publisher 1992; 249-275.

20. Gross S, Gee AP, Worthington-White DA, Eds: Progress in clinical and biological research, bone marrow purging and processing. Alan R.Liss Publisher 1990; Vol 333.

21. Gribben GJ, Freedman AS, Neuberg D, Roy DC, Blake KW, Woo SD, Grossbard ML, Rabinowe SN, Coral F, Freeman GJ, Ritz J, Nadler LM: Immunologic purging of marrow assessed by PCR before autologous bone marrow transplantation for B-cell lymphoma. N Engl J Med 1991; 325:1525-1533.

22. Moss TJ, Sanders DG: Detection of neuroblastoma cells in blood. J Clin Oncol 1990; 8:736-740.

23. To LB, Haylock DN, Dyson PG, Thorp D, Roberts MM, Juttner CA: An unusual pattern of hematopoietic reconstitution in patients with acute myeloid leukemia transplanted with autologous recovery phase peripheral blood. Bone Marrow Transplant 1990; 6:109-114.

24. Frame JN, Collins NH, Cartagena T, Waldman H, O'Reilly RJ, Dupont B, Kernan NA: T cell depletion of human bone marrow: comparison of Campath-1 plus complement, anti-T-cell ricin A chain immunotoxin and soybean agglutinin alone or in combination with sheep erythrocytes or immunomagnetic beads. Transplantation 1989; 47:984-988.

25. Keever CA, Small TN, Flomenberg N, Heller G, Pekle K, Black P, Pecora A, Gilio A, Kernan N, O'Reilly RJ: Immune reconstitution following bone marrow transplantation: comparison of recipients of T cell depleted marrow with recipients of conventional marrow grafts. Blood 1989; 73:1340-1350.

26. Lu L, Xiao M, Shen RN, Grigsby S, Broxmeyer HE: Enrichment, characterization, and responsiveness of single primitive CD34 human umbilical cord blood hematopoietic progenitors with high proliferative and replating potential.Blood 1993; 81:41-48.

27. Wagner JL, Broxmeyer HE, Byrd RL, Zehnbauer B, Schmeckpeper B, Shah N, Griffin C, Emanuel PD, Zuckerman KS, Cooper S, Carow C.Bias W, Santos GW: Transplantation of umbilical cord blood after myeloablative therapy. Analysis of engraftment. Blood 1992; 79:1874-

1881.

28. Vilmer E, Sterkers G, Rahimy C.Denamar E, Elion J, Broyart A, Lescocut B, JM, Gerota J, Blot P: HLA-mismatched cord blood transplantation in a patient with advanced leukemia. Transplantation 1992; 53:1155-1157.

29. Touraine JL: Transplantation of both fetal liver and thymus in severe combined immunodeficiency: Interaction between donor's and recipient's cells in fetal liver transplantation. Excerpta Med 1980; 514:277.

30. Meyers R, Good RA: Reconstitution of hematopoietic function in post-hepatic aplasia following high-dose cyclophosphamide and allogeneic fetal liver transplantation. Exp Hematol 1977; 5(Suppl 2):46.

31. Sharkis SJ, Santos GW, Colvin M: Elimination of acute myelogenous leukemia cells from marrow and tumor suspensions in the rat with 4-hydroperoxycyclophosphamide. Blood 1980; 55:521-523.

32. Labopin M, Gorin NC: Autologous bone marrow transplantation in 2502 patients with acute leukemia in Europe: a retrospective study. Leukemia 1992; 6(Suppl 4):95-99.

33. Filipovich AH, Vallera DA, Youle RJ, Quinones RR, Neville DM Jr, Kersey JH: Ex vivo treatment of donor bone marrow with anti-T-cell immunotoxins for prevention of graft-versus-host disease. Lancet 1984; 1:469-472.

34. Byers V, Henslee JP, Kernan NA, Blazar BR, Gingrich R, Phillips GL, LeMaistre CF, Gilliland G, Antin JH, Martin P, Tutscha PJ, Trown P, Ackerman SL, O'Reilly RJ, Scannon PJ: Use of an anti-pan T-lymphocyte ricin A chain immunotoxin in steroid-resistant acute graft-versus-host disease. Blood 1990; 75:1426-1432.

35. Neben S, Hemman S, Montgomery M, Ferrara J, Mauch P: Hematopoietic stem cell deficit of transplanted bone marrow previously exposed to cytoxic agents. Experimental Hematology 1993; 21:156-162.

36. Brenner, MK, Rill DR, Moen RC, Krance RA, Mirro J Jr, Anderson WF, Ihle JN: Gene-marking to trace origin of relapse after autologous bone-marrow transplantation.Lancet 1993; 341:85-86.

37. Bostrom B: Can maximal dose chemotherapy with marrow growth factors replace autologous bone marrow transplantation? In: Dicke KA, Armitage JO, Dicke-Evinger MJ, Eds. Proceedings of the fifth international symposium of Autologous BMT. Omaha, Nebraska: The University of Nebraska Medical Center Publisher 1991; 861-868.

38. Hryniuk WM, Levine MN: Analysis of dose intensity for adjuvant chemotherapy trials in stage II breast cancer. J Clin Oncol 1986; 4:1162-1170.

39. Levin L, Hryniuk WM: Dose intensity analysis of chemotherapy regimen in ovarian carcinoma. J Clin Oncol 1987; 5:756-767.

40. Jodrell DI, Egorin MJ, Canetta RM, Langenberg P, Goldbloom EP, Burroughs JN, Goodlow JL, Tan S, Wiltshaw E: Relationships between carboplatin exposure and tumor response and toxicity in patients with ovarian cancer. J of Clin Oncol 1992; 10:520-528.

41. Offit K, Burns JP, Cunningham I, Jhanwar SC, Black P, Kernan NA, O'Reilly RJ, Changanti RSK: Cytogenetic analysis of chimerism and leukemia relapse in chronic myelogenous leukemia patients after T cell-depleted bone marrow transplantation. Blood 1990; 75:1346-1355.

42. Goldman JM, Gale RP, Horowitz MM, Biggs JC, Champlin RE, Gluckman E, Hoffmann RG, Jacobsen SJ, Marmont AM, McGlave PB, Messner HA, Rimm AA, Rozman C, Speck B, Tura S, Weisner RS, Bortin MM: Bone marrow transplantation for chronic myelogenous leukemia in chronic phase: Increased risk of relapse associated with T-cell depletion. Ann Intern Med 1988; 108:806-814.

43. Schwarer AP, Jiang YZ, Brookes PA, Barret AJ, Batchelor JR, Goldman JM, Lechler RI: Frequency of anti-recipient alloreactive helper T-cell precursors in donor blood and graft-versus-host disease after HLA-identical sibling bone marrow transplantation. Lancet 1993; 341:203-204.

44. Mackinnon S, Barnett L, Bourhis JH, Black P, Heller G, O'Reilly RJ: Myeloid and lymphoid chimerism after T-cell-depleted bone marrow transplantation: Evaluation of conditioning regimens using the polymerase chain reaction to amplify human minisatellite regions of genomic DNA. Blood 1992; 80:3235-3241.

45. Kernan NA, Bordignon C, Keever CA, Cunningham I, Castro-Malaspina H, Collins NH, Small TN, Brochstein J, Emanuel D, Laver J, Shank B, Burns J, Flomenberg N, Gulati SC, Dupont B, O'Reilly RJ: Graft failures after T-cell depleted marrow transplants for leukemia: Clinical and in vitro characteristics. Transplantation Proceedings 1987; 19 (Suppl 7):29-32.

46. Patterson J, Prentice HG, Brenner MK, Gilmore M, Janossy G, Ivory K, Skeggs D, Morgan H, Lord J, Blacklock HA, Hoffbrand AV, Apperley JF, Goldman JM, Burnett A, Gribben J, Alcorn M, Pearson C, McVickers I, Hann IM, Reid C, Wardle D, Gravett PJ, Bacigalupo A, Robertson AG: Graft rejection following HLA matched T-lymphocyte depleted bone marrow transplantation. British J of Haematology 1986; 63:221-230.

47. Laurent G, Maraninchi D, Gluckman E, Vernant JP, Derocq JM, Gaspard MH, Rio B, Michalet M, Reiffers J, Dreyfus F, Casellas P, Schneider P, Blythman HE, Bouloux, Jansen FK: Donor bone marrow treatment with T101 Fab fragment-ricin A-chain immunotoxin prevents graft-versus-host disease. Bone Marrow Transplant 1989; 4:367-371.

48. Korngold R, Sprent J: T-cell subsets and graft-versus-host disease. Transplantation 1987; 44:335-339.

49. Soiffer RJ, Murray C, Mauch P, Anderson KC, Freedman AS, Rabinowe SN, Takvorian T, Robertson MJ, Spector N, Gonin R, Miller KB, Rudders RA, Freeman A, Blake K, Coral F, Nadler LM, Ritz J: Prevention of graft-versus-host disease by selective depletion of CD6-Positive T-lymphocytes from donor bone marrow. J of Clin Oncol 1992; 10:1191-1200.

50. Marmont AM, Horowitz MM, Gale RP, Sobocinski K, Ash RC, van Bekkum DW, Champlin RI, Dick KA, Goldman JM, Good RA, Herzig RH, Hong R, Masaoka T, Rimm AA, Ringden O, Speck B, Weiner RS, Bortin MM: T-cell depletion of HLA-identical transplants in leukemia. Blood 1991; 78:2120-2130.

51. Welte K, Ciobanu N, Moore MAS, Gulati SC, O'Reilly RJ, Mertelsmann R: Defective interleukin 2 production in patients after bone marrow transplantation and in vitro restoration of defective T-lymphocyte pro-

liferation by highly purified interleukin-2. Blood 1984; 64:380-385.

52. Sykes M, Romick ML, Sachs DH: Interleukin-2 prevents graft-versus-host disease while preserving the graft-versus-leukemia effect of allogeneic T-cells. Proc Natl Acad Sci 1990; 87:5633-5637.

53. Sullivan KM, Storb R, Buckner D, Fefer A, Fisher L, Weiden PL, Witherspoon RP, Appelbaum FR, Banaji M, Hansen J, Martin P, Sanders JE, Singer J, Thomas D: Graft-versus-host disease as adoptive immunotherapy in patients with advanced hematologic neoplasms. N Eng J Med 1989; 828-834.

54. Soiffer RJ, Murray C, Cochran K, Cameron C, Wang E, Schow PW, Daley JF, Ritz J: Clinical and immunologic effects of prolonged infusion of low-dose recombinant interleukin 2 after autologous and T-cell-depleted allogeneic bone marrow transplantation. Blood 1992; 79:517-526.

55. Antin JH, Ferrara JLM: Cytokine dysregulation and acute graft-versus-host disease. Blood 1992; 80:2964-2968.

56. Herve P, Wijdenes J, Bergerat JP, Bordigoni P, Milpied N, Cahn JY, Clement C, Beliard R, Morel-Fourrier B, Racadot E, Troussard X, Benz-Lemoine F, Gaud C, Legros M, Attal M, Kloft M, Peters A: Treatment of corticosteroid resistant acute graft-versus-host disease by in vivo administration of anti-interleukin-2 receptor monoclonal antibody (B-B10). Blood 1990; 75:1017-1023.

57. Higuchi CM, Thompson JA, Petersen FB, Buckner CD, Fefer A: Toxicity and immunomodulatory effects of interleukin-2 after autologous bone marrow transplantation for hematologic malignancies. Blood 1991; 77:2561-2568.

58. Ferrara JLM, Deeg HJ: Graft-versus-host disease. N Eng J Med 1991; 324:667-672.

59. Shapiro RS: Epstein-Barr Virus-Associated B-Cell lymphoproliferative disorders in immunodeficiency: Meeting the challenge. J Clin Oncol 1990; 8:371-373.

CHAPTER 2

TECHNIQUES OF EX VIVO MANIPULATION

Purging methods should ensure complete hematopoietic engraftment without causing undue recurrence of the malignancy. The purging techniques can either utilize positive selection in which the hematopoietic cells are enriched and used for hematopoietic reconstitution, or use negative selection in which the malignant cells are preferentially eliminated from the stem cell harvest (Table 1).

METHODS USED TO PROVE THE ROLE OF PURGING

Several approaches are utilized to decide which methods to use for purging. Most often the efficacy of the approach is first determined in an animal model system.[1-2] Subsequently, the techniques are tried in preclinical malignant cell line models or occasionally directly carried out to phase I patient trial.[3-34] Throughout the text, animal models used for proving the role of purging will be detailed.

Assessment of ex vivo purging of malignant cells is often difficult and subject to error as the patient may behave different than the immortalized cell lines, for example, most of the B-lymphoid cell lines have the EBV genome integrated into the DNA. Certain cancers do not grow in currently available culture media and at times fresh cancer cells can grow in vitro. Therefore, for each type of cancer an appropriate model has to be selected. Some of the cancer cell lines can grow colonies on soft agar or methylcellulose. In such cases, decrease in the number of colonies can be used as an index of purging benefit. The data can be further improved by plating concentrate of treated cells.[33] Most experiments are performed by growing cells in liquid culture and scoring the number of cells after treatment. Such analysis can be performed immediately or by 7-21 days in culture. In some situations, malignant cells emerge above the lower limits of detection in a few days and extrapolating the data can give a good approximation of the benefit of purging (Figure 1).[34] In this figure, greater than 4 logs of cytotoxicity was observed. In vivo conditions can be simulated by spiking the malignant cells with irradiated bone marrow. The toxicity to the hematopoietic stem cells can be quantitated by adding irradiated cancer cells to the reaction and evaluating the toxicity towards CFU-GM, BFU-e and CFU-GM.

Table 1. Hematopoietic stem cell purging

Positive selection
    Antibody
        Cell sorter
    Panning
        Avidin-biotin immunoabsorption columns
    Long-term stem cell culture
Negative selection
    Antibody
        Complement-mediated cytolysis
        Magnetic bead conjugation
        Toxin conjugation
        Immunorosettes
    Biochemical
        Cytotoxic drugs with or without enhancers
    Biophysical
        Lectin agglutination
        Counter flow elutriation
        Adsorption columns
        Phototherapy
    Biologic
        Interleukin-2, lymphokine activated killer cells,
        Interferons
        Differentiation agents
        Anti-sense oligodeoxynucleotides

Figure 1. Dose response of leukemic cell lines to MC-540. Ten million cells were incubated with different doses of MC-540 at 37°C and simultaneously exposed to white light at 50,000 1x for 1h, then washed twice with RPMI 1640 and kept in long-term culture for up to 20 days. Bars, standard deviation; REH, a lymphoblastic leukemia cell line. Reproduced with permission from Cancer Research.[34]

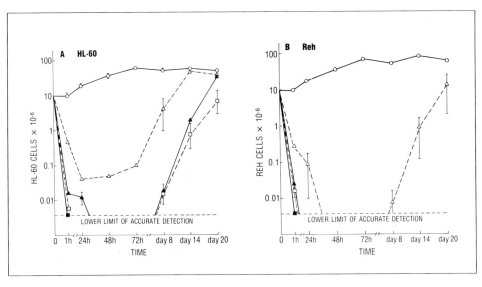

Various models are available to predict the synergistic or antagonistic effect of combining different purging methods. One useful method was described by Chou and Talalay.[35] Analyzing interaction of multiple drug effects by this method has several important features: (a) it utilizes small numbers of data points; (b) it quantitates synergism, summation or antagonism at different effect levels; (c) it provides information about relative potency of each drug and their mixtures; (d) it determines the sigmoidicity of the dose-effect curve, exclusive drug effects and includes these parameters into the overall calculations. Many of these features are not available by the isobologram or the fractional product methods. Furthermore, the availability of computer software of this method greatly facilitates the analysis.[35] Combination of 4-HC and VP-16 at a 4-HC: VP-16 drug ratio of 1:0.342 was found to be the best for selective toxicity towards HL-60 cells and was superior to the "4-HC, adriamycin" or "VP-16, adriamycin" combination for usefulness in purging bone marrow (Figure 2).[36]

In the rat leukemia model of Hagenbeek et al,[1] animals that were susceptible to acute promyelocytic leukemia were injected with different numbers of leukemic cells to evaluate how many leukemic cells are needed to develop leukemia. It was found that the median dose, i.e., 50% of the rats die at this level, of the leukemic cells in the rat model was 25 cells. In human beings, this median dose would correspond to approximately 3500 leukemic cells. Considering most BMTs are performed when the bone marrow is in remission, this model would imply that approximately 15 to 150 leukemic cells are being infused into the patient. The risk of leukemia relapse would be between 1% and 5% according to this theoretical model. Therefore, several authors believe that it is more important to emphasize the role of the conditioning regimen of the patient rather than be concerned about the relatively small amount of leukemia remaining in the bone marrow. The proof that leukemic cells can be specifically purged from the bone marrow with cytotoxic drug (4-hydroperoxycyclophosphamide [4-HC]) was established in the rat model system. 4-HC has since been used in several purging protocols.[2-4]

POSITIVE SELECTION

STEM CELL-SPECIFIC ANTIBODY

CD-33 and CD-34 antigens are expressed on early hematopoietic stem cells, but unfortunately leukemic blasts and few other cells express these antigens.[5-7] Several investigators are developing methods to enrich the HSCs. Concentrating hematopoietic progenitors from autologous peripheral blood stem cells or marrow would overcome many of the complications described below. Ability to work with a highly enriched fraction of progenitor cells for cryopreservation that is free of cellular debris and unwanted cells such as granulocytes and platelets should reduce the risk of clot formation after thawing. Furthermore, the clinical side effects due to the unwanted cellular debris, such as fever, pulmonary embolism and respiratory failure will be reduced. The hematopoietic progenitor cell population concentrated from marrow should be essentially free of red blood cells, as this will eliminate hemolytic complications. Since progenitors make up less than 1% of marrow, concentrating them should significantly reduce the volume of stem cells to be frozen, thus decreasing the amount of DMSO required and therefore reducing the possibility of harmful side effects of DMSO. The reduced volume of concentrated hematopoietic progenitors compared to whole autologous marrow should also facilitate the freezing process as well as contribute to more uniform freezing of the progenitor cells and require less space for marrow storage. Specifically isolating the hematopoietic progenitors responsible for engraftment would also provide a population essentially depleted of tumor

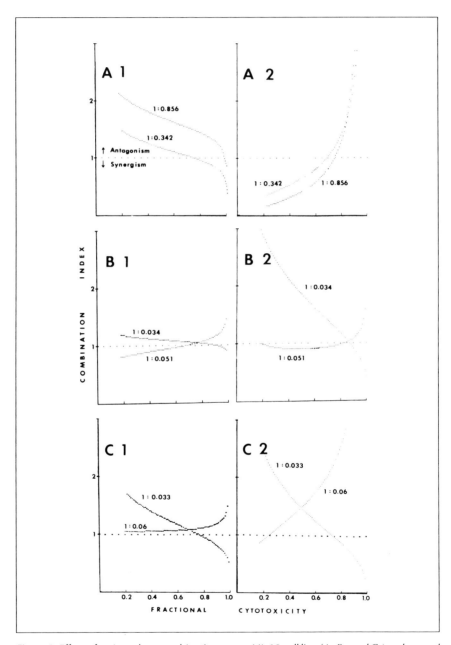

Figure 2. Effect of various drug combinations upon HL-60 cell line (A$_1$,B$_1$, and C$_1$) and normal BM CFU-GM (A$_2$, B$_2$, and C$_2$). A, 4-HC:VP-16; B, 4-HC:ADR. C, VP-16:ADR. Data points above the horizontal dotted line, antagonism; data points below the horizontal dotted line, synergism. Reproduced with permission from Cancer Research.[36]

cells. Furthermore, gene transfer studies will have a significantly improved homogenous cell population to work with. To be clinically useful, a device designed to isolate marrow progenitor cells must have sufficient capacity to process the large number of whole marrow cells (>10 billion) required for autologous marrow transplantation. The device should be simple and economical to operate. It must be nontoxic and yield highly reproducible results following each cell separation procedure. The capacity to concentrate progenitors and remove these unwanted cell populations can be measured experimentally in the laboratory.

Investigators have attempted to concentrate hematopoietic progenitors by exploiting differences in size and density between these cells and other marrow elements. Centrifugation has been the major approach used in these separation procedures. The methods usually involve a density gradient to separate the mononuclear cell layer, which contains the progenitors, from the granulocytes and red blood cells. Most clinical methods have used Ficoll-Hypaque, while some investigators have utilized Ficoll-metrizoate or Percoll as density gradient media.[4,9] Losses of up to 50% of the mononuclear cells as well as toxic effects of the density gradient media on marrow progenitors have been observed by using these technologies. Delayed engraftment after transplantation has also been documented. The recent development of monoclonal antibodies that identify hematopoietic progenitors has generated interest in procedures that can specifically isolate these antibody-labeled cells from marrow. A number of technologies have been used for positive selection of cells labeled with monoclonal antibodies. The fluorescence activated cell sorter (FACS) has been used for the isolation of hematopoietic progenitors for research work, but is impractical for sorting more than a few million cells. The "panning technique" in which cells are separated on plastic petri dishes coated with antibodies, is relatively uncomplicated but produces variable yield and purity of the captured cells and is also cumbersome to use for large scale selection procedures.[10]

Magnetic immunoselection has recently been utilized for cell separation.[11,12] In this technology, cells are first labeled with antibody-coated paramagnetic microspheres and then a magnetic device is used to separate labeled from unlabeled cells. This technique has been used clinically with antibodies directed to remove tumor cells from the marrow. For positive selection, chymopapain is usually required to digest the antigen and to release the cells. Recently, a specific enzyme that digests CD-34 Ag has become available and will allow wider application of this technique. Investigations are ongoing to see if this approach can be used for positive selection.[13]

Immunoadsorption column devices can be used for positive as well as negative cell selection. However, most of the technologies described above rely on the relatively weak binding (dissociation constant = 10^{-8} to 10^{-9} M) between cell surface antigen and antibody on the solid phase surface, and thus require incubation of cells to attach to the solid phase surface. Indirect immunoadsorption devices employing ligands such as Protein A, plant ligands, fluorescein isothiocyanate, or goat anti-mouse antisera have been used to bind antibody labeled cells. Methods are being developed to properly utilize these approaches and concentrate the hematopoietic stem cell with minimal contamination of other cells; especially the tumor cells. Berenson et al have developed an immunoadsorption technique that relies on the high affinity interaction between the protein avidin and the vitamin biotin (dissociation constant = 10^{-15} M).[14,15] Cells are first labeled with a mouse monoclonal antibody to the antigen of interest and then treated with a biotin-conjugated anti-mouse antibody. Treated cells are then passed (without incubation) through a column of avidin-coated beads. Antibody-labeled cells adhere to the beads and nonlabeled cells pass through the column. Bound cells are subsequently removed by mechanical agitation of the beads in the column. Without incubation, nonspecific binding is minimized and greater than 10^{10} cells can be separated in a short time period. This technique has been successfully used for enriching CD-34 positive cells from bone marrow and peripheral blood.[18]

The avidin-biotin immunoabsorption column was originally used in a model system to remove up to three logs of Daudi lymphoma cells from human marrow. Initial studies also demonstrated that T cells could be eliminated from peripheral blood using this device and this approach can be useful for allogeneic BMT. Several laboratories have developed monoclonal antibodies MY10, 12.8 and BI-3C5, that recognize a 115,000 dalton glycoprotein (CD-34) present on 1-3% of human marrow cells, including immature blast cells, but minimally (usually not detectable) expressed on mature cells in marrow including lymphocytes, granulocytes, red blood cells, and platelets.[5-7] Further studies have shown that the CD-34 antigen is found on virtually all committed hematopoietic progenitors that are measured in assays of colony-forming cells including erythroid progenitors (BFU-e), granulocyte-monocyte progenitors (CFU-GM), and progenitors that give rise to mixed lineage colonies (CFU-Mix). Precursors of colony-forming cells that grow in long-term marrow culture were also found to be CD-34 positive, suggesting that more primitive progenitor cell populations also expressed this antigen.[8]

Immunophenotyping studies have been performed to test the reactivity of the anti-CD-34 antibody 12.8 with malignant cells. Marrow cells from patients with multiple myeloma and acute leukemia were tested by immunofluorescence and FACS analysis, while lymphomas and solid tumors were evaluated by using an immunoperoxidase technique on tissue samples. These studies showed that antibody 12.8 does not react with tumor cells from patients with lymphomas, myeloma and most solid tumors including breast cancer and neuroblastoma. Tumor cells from many patients with leukemia and some patients with lung cancer showed reactivity with the 12.8 antibody. Watt et al[16] have reported similar findings with antibody BI-3C5, which also identifies the CD-34 antigen, demonstrating its lack of reactivity with both Hodgkin's and non-Hodgkin's lymphomas and the majority of solid tumors. Therefore, hematopoietic progenitors can be enriched with use of anti-CD-34 antibody. Five lethally irradiated baboons were given CD-34+ (bone marrow devoid of detectable mature and immature T and B lymphocytes) allogeneic BMT. All animals engrafted with donor cells by cytogenetic analysis. Three animals died of infections 34, 43 and 109 days after transplant. The other two animals had donor erythroid, granulocytic and monocytic engraftment. This study suggests that CD-34+ enriched cells will probably be useful in human allogeneic BMT.[17]

CD-34 positive cells have been enriched using avidin-biotin binding collums (Cellpro Inc.). Shpall et al have shown that CD-34 enriched mononuclear cells are capable of hematopoietic engraftment after high dose cyclo-phosphamide, cisplatinum and BCNU therapy. The first cohort of nine patients (breast cancer 6, NHL3) received CD-34+ cells alone. The second cohort of nine breast cancer patients received CD-34+ cells plus 16 mcg/kg G-CSF intravenously daily over 4 hours for 21 days post-AUBMT. The patients achieved a granulocyte count of >500/mm^3 and an unsupported platelet count >20,000/mm^3, respectively, at a mean of 21 and 17 days post-AUBMT for cohort 1, and 11 and 16 days post-AUBMT for cohort 2. No late graft failures have occurred to date (longest follow-up, 7 months).[18] Evaluation of immune function in the first seven patients revealed normal natural killer cell and cytolytic T cell activity within 4 to 8 weeks following CD-34+ infusion. Granulocyte recovery was significantly shortened in pa-tients who received CD-34+ cells plus G-CSF, compared to patients who received CD-34+ cells alone (p=0.031). Future experiments are investigating the role of G-CSF primed, CD-34+ peripheral blood cells in AUSCT.

STEM CELL CULTURE

Hematopoiesis can be maintained for several weeks in vitro in long-term bone marrow culture (LTBMC). Under certain culture conditions, growth of hematopoietic cells appears to be dependent upon the establishment of an adherent feeder layer derived from marrow stromal cells. Usually, the prolif-eration of tumor cells is not favored in this system, and in general, normal hematopoietic cells appear to have a selective growth advantage over the neoplastic clones. Recently, LTBMC have been used as a source of normal bone marrow (BM) progenitors for reconstitution of hematopoiesis after myeloablative chemoradiotherapy in patients with acute myeloid leukemia (AML) and chronic myelogenous leukemia (CML). In addition, LTBMC has been proposed as a method of in vitro purging for patients with acute lymphoid leukemia (ALL) and multiple myeloma.[19-23]

Although adequate hematopoietic reconstitution has occurred following the infusion of stem cells grown in LTBMC, poor growth from most patients, fungal and bacterial contamination and major loss of BM progenitors are some concerns that arise from culturing the marrow for the time required (10-25 days) for the disappearance of tumor cells. In order to improve upon the above problems, attempts were made to grow hematopoietic progenitors in plastic gas-permeable bags with and without the addition of selected hematopoietic colony-stimulating factors (CSFs), i.e., interleukin 1 (IL-1) and interleukin 3 (IL-3). Mononuclear cells in bags treated with IL-1 alone demonstrated only transient beneficial effects, and the number of hematopoi-etic precursors fell below the level of cells observed in the control bag during the culture. IL-1 and IL-3 induced 1.8- and 5.3-fold peak increases in BFU-e and CFU-GM at weeks 1 and 4, respectively. Simultaneous flow cytometric analysis of CD-34+/CD-33+ cells and DNA content showed increased num-bers and proliferation of the committed BM progenitors when CSFs were added to the bag. These results indicate that long-term production of hema-topoietic cells can be sustained in the absence of a feeder layer in plastic gas-permeable bags, and that stimulation with CSFs induces a higher recovery of BM progenitors, while the longevity of hematopoiesis is not altered.[24] Several cytokines have been recently evaluated for ex vivo expansion of CD-34 positive cells. In one such study, avidin-biotin column separated CD-34 positive cells (Cell pro columns) were expanded with hematopoietic growth factors (IL-1, IL-3 and c-kit ligand also called stem cell factor). Synergistic amplification of total cells and progenitor cells was observed with 223-fold expansion of total cells and 109-fold expansion of progenitors when all three factors were used together. The growth of peripheral blood cells was several fold better than that of bone marrow.[25] Improvements in these approaches may reduce the amount of cells which need to be harvested for transplantation and may decrease the duration of cytopenia after transplant. Further research in expansion of hematopoietic progenitors will also allow markedly improved methods for allogeneic BMT and genetic engineering.[26,27]

NEGATIVE SELECTION

ANTIBODIES

Several antibodies have been selected for clinical trials and have shown preferential binding to the malignant cell and cytotoxicity with the use of complement, toxins and radioactive molecules. Furthermore, the antibodies are also used to separate cells by physical methods (immunomagnetic, avidin-biotin columns). Specific antibodies are available for small cell lung cancer and neuroblastoma.[4,9,11,12] Antibodies with preferential binding to acute myeloblastic leukemia (AML) and acute lymphoblastic leukemia (ALL) are also in clinical trials.

Significant data has now been published with regards to improving the purging of T-lymphocytes.[28-30] Immunomagnetic separation methods have been developed and are now entering meaningful clinical trials. In one such approach, immunomagnetic separation procedure using an avidin-based magnetic affinity cobalt colloid was used. Bone marrow cells were incubated with a combination of four antibodies against T cells (CD2, CD3, CD4 and CD8). The cells were washed and then incubated with the biotinylated, affinity-purified IgG fraction of goat anti-mouse immunoglobulins followed by an avidin-based magnetic affinity colloid. The cells were then run through a high-magnetic gradient separation column utilizing an external samarium cobalt magnet. The number of residual T-lymphocytes was assessed by limiting dilutin analysis of clonogenic T-lymphocytes. This procedure produces an approximately 1.7-log reduction of antibody-reactive cells with 45% recovery of hematopoietic progenitors (granulocyte-macrophage colony-forming cells, (CFU-GM).[28] This causes a reduction of T-lymphocytes in the bone marrow graft to approximately 5×10^5 cells/kg body weight. Allogeneic BMT after selective removal of CD 5 and/or CD 8 positive lymphocytes is now ongoing. (See also Chapter 4.)

BIOCHEMICAL

Several drugs have been evaluated for purging hematopoietic stem cells (HSC). 4-HC is the most extensively evaluated. (See also Chapter 1.) Although 4-HC is cytotoxic to normal early hematopoietic progenitors (Figure 3),[31] most studies have found it to be significantly more toxic to tumor cells especially lymphoma, nonlymphoblastic leukemia, breast cancer, neuroblastoma and Ewing's sarcoma cells.[32-36] In one early trial,[32] patients with relapsed lymphoma or acute leukemia in complete remission received autologous bone marrow transplants purged with increasing doses of 4-HC. Buffy coat frac-

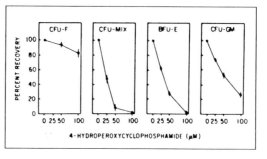

Figure 3. Comparison of the effect of 4-HC on human marrow stomal and hematopoietic progenitor cells. Marrow cells were incubated with 4-HC, washed and then assayed for fibroblast (CFU-F), mixed (CFU-Mix), erythroid (BFU-e), and granulocyte-macrophage (CFU-GM) colony-forming cells. Values shown are the mean ± 0.9; BFU-e, 98 ± 26; CFU-GM, 79 ± 23; CFU-F, 91 ± 11. Note that CFU-F are relatively resistant to 4-HC as compared with CFU-Mix, BFU-e, and CFU-GM. Reproduced with permission from Blood.[31]

tions of the marrow were treated with 4-HC at nucleated cell concentrations of 2×10^7 cells/ml for 30 minutes at 37°C and the treated marrows were frozen with dimethylsulfoxide in the liquid phase of nitrogen. All 26 patients transplanted with marrow purged with 40-100 mcg/ml of 4-HC engrafted. There was a suggestion of a dose-response relationship between 4-HC dose and hematologic recovery: the median time to 500 granulocytes per microliter was 14 days in the patients treated at 40 mcg/ml of 4-HC versus 24 days in the patients treated at 100 mcg/ml. Three of ten patients who received bone marrow treated with 4-HC at 120 mcg/ml failed to show any evidence of hematologic recovery by day 21 after BMT and were given their back-up marrow; one of these patients subsequently engrafted and two died without evidence of engraftment. Based on these results, 100 mcg/ml was chosen as the dose of 4-HC to be used in the subsequent autologous BMT studies, although lack of any evidence of engraftment by day 21 after 4-HC-purged autologous BMT would not currently be considered graft failure. However, experience at other institutions found 4-HC to be markedly more toxic to the normal hematopoietic elements and new institutions planning to use 4-HC should do their own preclinical studies.[33,36] One reason for this variation may be the amount of red cells contaminating the mononuclear cells. Red cells contain aldehyde dehydrogenase; an important mechanism of cellular resistance to cyclophosphamide, which oxidizes 4-HC to the inactive carboxyphosphamide form.[37] Some of the relative resistance of hematopoietic stem cells and other normal cells to cyclophosphamide may result from their high levels of aldehyde dehydrogenase. Aldehyde dehydrogenase also appears to be an important mechanism for tumor cells resistant to cyclophosphamide. To decrease the variability in 4-HC cytotoxicity resulting from the variable red cell content of the incubation mixture, some investigators remove red cells from the marrow graft prior to purging by density-gradient separation. With little red cell contamination of the incubation mixture to inhibit 4-HC, the dose of 4-HC for clinical purging has been decreased from 100 mcg/ml to 60 mcg/ml at one institution. Other institutions custom dose 4-HC by doing pre-purging evaluation to decide the dose which gives 50% toxicity towards CFU-GM.[32] The effects of 4-HC on the hematopoietic and stromal elements of human bone marrow have been evaluated (Figure 3). The data suggests that the early hematopoietic progenitors are spared by 4-HC.[31] Marrow cells were exposed to 4-HC and then assayed for mixed (CFU-Mix), erythroid

(BFU-e), granulo-monocytic (CFU-GM), and marrow fibroblast (CFU-F) colony-forming cells and studied in the long-term marrow culture (LTMC) system. The inhibition of colony formation by 4-HC was dose and cell-concentration dependent. The cell most sensitive to 4-HC was CFU-Mix [ID_{50} (50% inhibitory dose) 31 mcmol/L] followed by BFU-e (ID_{50} 41 mcmol). CFU-GM (ID_{50} 89 mcmol), and CFU-F (ID_{50} 235 mcmol). In LTMC, a dose-related inhibition of CFU-GM production was noted. Marrow treated with 300 mcmol 4-HC were completely depleted of CFU-GM, but were able to generate these progenitors in LTMC. Marrow stromal progenitors giving rise to stromal layers in LTMC, although less sensitive to 4-HC cytotoxicity, were damaged by 4-HC also in a dose-related manner. Marrow treated with 4-HC up to 300 mcmol, gave rise to stromal layers composed of fibroblasts, endothelial cells, adipocytes, and macrophages. Cocultivation experiments with freshly isolated autologous hematopoietic cells showed that stromal layers derived from 4-HC treated marrow were capable of sustaining the long-term production of CFU-GM as well as controls. These results indicate that: (1) Hematopoietic progenitors cells, CFU-Mix, BFU-e, and CFU-GM, are highly sensitive to 4-HC, whereas marrow stromal progenitor cells are relatively resistant. (2) Marrow treated with 300 mcmol 4-HC that are depleted of CFU-Mix, BFU-e, and CFU-GM can generate CFU-GM in LTMC, suggesting that most primitive hematopoietic stem cells (not represented by CFU-Mix) are spared by 4-HC up to this dose.[31] Other investigators have similar results[32] and therefore, the above colony assays need to be evaluated with caution for predicting pluripotent stem cell survival after 4-HC treatment in vitro. It appears that natural killer (NK) cells are involved in the control of hematopoiesis. Cardoso et al[38] have assayed NK cell activity from human bone marrow (BM) following "purge" with 4-HC at 60 mcg/ml for 30 min in vitro. In all cases studied, lytic activity against the K562 cell line was either significantly decreased or abolished following 4-HC purge. Although NK activity was significantly affected by 4-HC treatment, no major differences in the phenotype between the purged and unpurged population were seen. Furthermore, while in vitro culture of BM with IL-2 resulted in a significant increment of NK activity, no IL-2 responsive cells were found in the 4-HC purged BM after 14 days of culture. This data suggests that pharmacological purging of bone marrow results in a persistent functional decline of NK cell activity and may serve as a useful model for the study of the ontogeny of NK cells and may have implications regarding relapse of disease after 4-HC purged transplantation. Early investigations have shown the efficacy of cyclophosphamide in treating many different malignancies. (See Chapter 4.)

VP-16, a podophyllotoxin derivative, is now often a part of the standard treatment of human lymphomas or leukemias; it produces metaphase arrest and inhibits cells from entering mitosis. In addition, VP-16 may act synergistically with an alkylating agent because of its inhibitory activity on topoisomerase II, an enzyme that enhances DNA repair. VP-16 has also shown significant promise in purging and some investigators utilize combinations of VP-16 and 4-HC.[39-41] (See also Chapter 1.) Considering that 4-HC is not widely available, alternate drugs for purging were also evaluated.[9,33,40,41] For example, a mixture of nitrogen mustard and VP-16 is also highly effective in eliminating 3 to 4 logs of leukemia (K-562, HL-60) cells.[40]

BIOPHYSICAL

Proper use of flow cytometry or density gradient separation and exploitation of cell membrane difference can help design purging methods. Unfortunately, bulk processing is a problem and clinical application has been cumbersome. There are various machines available to help enrich mononuclear cells, e.g., removal of erythrocytes and platelets, so they can subsequently be purged by other methods (antibodies, drugs, etc.). Concomitant use of such separation can lower the cost and provide further reliability to the purging methods.[9,25,42-44]

Significant results have also been obtained in the preclinical experiments using lysosomotrophic agents which are preferentially cytotoxic towards leukemic cells.[45,46] Furthermore, ether lipids (ALP) have shown toxicity towards drug resistant malignant cell lines. In one recent study, ALP showed differential toxicity to neoplastic cells. It was determined that the effect of ALP on human myeloma cell lines are noted even when resistance to different chemotherapeutic agents had developed. The cell lines included RPMI 8226/s, 8226/Dox$_{40}$ (doxorubicin), 8226/LR$_5$ (melphalan), 8226/MR$_{40}$ (mitoxantrone), and 8226/DoxV (doxorubicin/verapamil). After exposure to ALP (50 mcg/ml), both the 8226/S and the drug resistant cell lines had significant toxicity in the first 4 hours with little additional kill after 24 hours. ALP (25 mcg/ml, 24 hr, 37°C) was highly effective against all cell lines showing the following percent depletion: 8226/S (99.89; n=5), 8226/LR$_5$ (99.84; n=6), 8226/Dox$_{40}$ (99.41; n=3), 8226/MR$_{40}$ (99.93; n=1). Mean log kills ranged from 2.3 to 3.9.[45] These results suggest that ALP may be an effective purging agent for patients with leukemia and multiple myeloma.

PHOTOTHERAPY

Several compounds sensitize cancer cells and specifically rupture cell membranes when exposed to light.[47-51] To assess the potential of photoradiation therapy for the in vitro purging of residual tumor cells prior to the stem cells use for AUBMT's, we studied normal marrow and tumor cell clonogenicity in response to different light-activated compounds by using the fluorescent dyes dihematoporphyrin ether (DHE) and merocyanine-540. After photoradiation of cells with white light, both DHE and merocyanine-540 showed high cytocidal activity toward lymphoid and myeloid neoplastic cells but had a significantly lesser effect on normal granulocyte-macrophage colony-forming units (CFU-GM), erythroid burst-forming units (BFU-e), and mixed colony-forming (CFU-GEMM) progenitor cells. Acute promyelocytic leukemia (HL-60), non-B, non-T, CALLA-positive acute lymphoblastic leukemia (Reh), and diffuse histiocytic B-cell lymphoma (SK-DHL-2) cell lines were exposed to different drug concentrations in combination with white light at a constant illumination rate of 50,000 lux. With DHE doses varying from 2.0 to 2.5 mcg/mL and merocyanine-540 concentrations from 14 to 20 mcg/mL, clonogenic tumor cells could be reduced by more than 4 logs when treated alone or in mixtures with normal irradiated human marrow cells. However, preferential cytotoxicity toward neoplastic cells was highly dependent on the mode of light activation. Merocyanine-540 had no substantial effect on malignant lymphoid (SK-DHL-2), and myeloid (HL-60) cells and on normal marrow myeloid precursors (CFU-GM) when drug incubation was performed in the dark and followed by light exposure of washed cells. Equal doses of merocyanine-540 (15 to 20 mcg/mL) could preferentially eliminate tumor cells under conditions of simultaneous light and drug treatment (30 min at 37°C). When using DHE (2.5 mcg/mL) with sequential drug and light exposure of cells, 29.3%, 46.8%, and 27.5% of normal marrow CFU-GM, BFU-e and CFU-GEMM were spared, respectively, whereas simultaneous treatment reduced both normal (CFU-GM) and neoplastic cells below the lower limit of detection (Figure 4).[48] These results indicate the usefulness of various photoradiation models for the ex vivo treatment of leukemic and lymphomatous bone marrow autografts. Conditions have to be optimized to

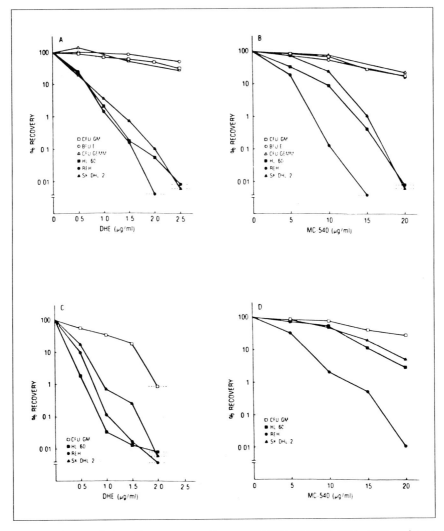

Figure 4. Photoradiation effects on normal human BM CFU-GM (□), BFU-e (○), and CFU-GEMM (△) as compared with clonogenic growth reduction of HL-60 (■), Reh (●), and SK-DHL-2 (▲) cells. (A) DHE/sequential drug-light treatment. (B) MC-540/simultaneous drug-light treatment. (C) DHE/simultaneous drug-light treatment. (D) MC-540/sequential drug-light treatment. Mean values from three or more separate experiments are given as the percentage of control (photoradiation in the abscence of DHE or MC-540;—— represents the lower limits of accurate detection as calculated from control experiments. Reproduced with permission from Blood.[48]

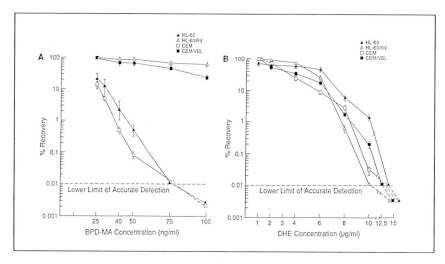

Figure 5. Cytotoxic activity of BPD-MA (A) and DHE (B) on HL-60 and CEM cell lines and their MDR+ drug-resistant sublines. (▲) HL-60; (△) HL-60/RV; (□) CEM; (■) CEM/VBL. Cells were concentrated at 2 x 10⁷/mL. Tumor cells were mixed with irradiated mononuclear light-density BM cells. Mean values from three or more separate experiments are given as the percentage of control samples (photoexposure in absence of BPD-MA or DHE). Reproduced with permission from Blood.[50]

utilize these compounds. Merocyanine-540 is already in phase I clinical trials. Sensitivity to phototherapeutic agents may persist even when the cancer cells have developed drug resistance to cytotoxic chemicals (Figure 5).[50]

BIOLOGICAL METHODS

Interleukin-2, lymphokine activated killer cells, and interferons have shown significant promise for purging HSC in pre-clinical evaluation.[49,52,53] In one study, the sensitivity of human myeloma (plasma cell leukemia) toward autologous and allogeneic lymphokine-activated killer (LAK) cells was evaluated.[54] Fresh plasma cell leukemia (PCL)-derived peripheral blood mononuclear cells (PBMC) and PBMC from three normal donors were cultured in the presence of recombinant interleukin-2 (rIL2; 1,000 U/ml) for subsequent use as cytotoxic effectors against fresh and continuously cultured myeloma cells. Target cell lysis was measured in a 4-hour[51]Cr radioisotope release assay. At an effector to target (E:T) ratio of 50:1, rIL2-induced PCL-PBMC lysed 48 ± 19% (mean ± 1 SD) of autologous myeloma targets, as compared to 89 ± 5, 95 ± 15, and 100 ± 9% lysis of standard LAK-sensitive Daudi cells (a standard control) and allogeneic myeloma cell lines SKO-007, and RPMI-8226, respectively. Normal PBMC-derived rIL2-induced (LAK) cells exhibited a slightly lower cytotoxic reactivity against allogeneic targets (61 ± 9, 60 ± 6, AND 81 ± 8% cytolysis of SKO-007, RPMI-8226, and Daudi cells, respectively, at a 50:1 E:T ratio). Cytotoxicity against myeloma (PCL) of autologous PCL-derived killer cells could be significantly (at least two-fold) enhanced when rIL-2 induced effector cells were preincubated for 18 hours in the presence of recombinant Interferon-α (rIFN-α:1,000 U/ml). These results indicate the potential antitumor efficacy of rIL2- an rIL2+ rIFN-α-activated killer cells in human myeloma (PCL). Further evaluation of

4-HC and VP-16 in combination with LAK cells were also evaluated for purging of myeloma cells. Myeloma cell lines (SK-RCS-1, RPMI-8226), lymphoma cell line (SK-DHL-2) and normal bone marrow (BM) cells were treated at different concentrations of 4-HC, VP-16. In separate experiments, LAK cells or antibodies were also used to treat the above cell lines. Clonogenic tumor cells from all three cell lines could be reduced by more than 4 logs when treated alone or as a mixture with irradiated normal bone marrow cells at a 4-HC concentration of 60 mcmol. Under similar conditions, approximately 1% of normal BM myeloid progenitor granulocyte-macrophage colony forming cells (CFU-GM) survived. Similar results were also obtained with LAK cells and antibodies.[54]

It is also possible that bone marrow can be mixed with various agents that cause differentiation of the malignant cell with eventual death of the cancer cell.[52,55,56] In this regard, the recent use of antisense oligodeoxynucleotides to selectively suppress Ph clone can be effectively utilized to purge Ph cells.[57] Recently, it has been shown that in some malignancies with specific genetic changes, the programmed cell death (apoptosis) is delayed. For example, in mammals, bcl-2 gene can prevent the death of myeloid or neuronal cells that occurs after withdrawal of certain growth factors, but it cannot protect cells from being killed by cytotoxic T-cells. Inhibition of cell death by improperly regulated expression of bcl-2 may be oncogenic, and may account for the follicular lymphomas seen with bcl-2 rearrangements and t(14:18) translocation.[56] Purging methods which alter the control mechanisms of apoptosis (including the use of growth factors) will have a major role in improving the success of BMT.[55-57]

COMBINED THERAPY

Several investigators have explored the approach of combined purging techniques with promising results.[58,59] Use of radioprotectants, e.g., WR 2721, may alter the efficiency of purging conditions.[60] In one recent study, four different purging methods were compared using a promyelocytic human cell line HL-60 and myeloid leukemic progenitor cells [colony-forming unit-leukemic (CFU-L)] from patients with acute myelogenous leukemia (AML). The antileukemic effect of (1) Single-cycle complement-mediated lysis by two different monoclonal antibodies (MoAbs) [M195 (CD33) and F23 (CD13) 40 mcg/mL], reactive with distinct antigens found on early myeloid cells and monocytes, used alone and in combinations; (2) 4-HC (80 mcmol or 100 mcmol) alone; or (3) combined with VP-16 (5 mcg/mL and (4) a cocktail of 1 through 3 as above (combined immuno-chemotherapy). More than 4 logs of HL-60 tumor cell elimination were observed after 1 hour of incubation with both MoAbs plus 4-HC + VP-16 while the single treatment (immunotherapy or chemotherapy) provided 1.5 and 3.5 logs of colony-forming inhibition, respectively. When the same protocols were tested on cryopreserved leukemic cells from eight patients with AML, CFU-L inhibition of 92.3%, 95.5%, and 99% was observed. MoAbs and 4-HC + VP-16 produced more than 3-log reduction of CFU-L colony formation. By comparison, the mean recovery of committed normal bone marrow progenitors after incubation with MoAbs and complement was 12% for CFU-granulocyte-macrophage (CFU-GM), 22.9% for burst-forming unit erythroid (BFU-e), and the recovery following 4-HC + VP-16 treatment was 4.4% for CFU-

GM and 5.6% BFU-e. In subsequent experiments, highly purified CD-34 blast cells, enriched by positive selection, and stimulated in liquid culture by cytokines (interleukin-1 [IL-1], IL-3, and combination of both) or MO-conditioned medium (MoCM), demonstrated that immunochemotherapy spares hematopoietic colony-forming progenitor cells in vitro.[8]

"Medicine is an art." —Angeli Gulati

The following chapters will describe how the techniques described above are being utilized in clinical trials. The results and future directions are also detailed.

REFERENCES

1. Hagenbeek A, Schultz FW, Martens ACM: In vitro or in vivo treatment of leukemia to prevent a relapse after autologous bone marrow transplantation. In: Dicke KA, Spitzer G, Jagannath S, eds. Autologous bone marrow transplantation: Proceedings of the Fourth International Symposium. MD Anderson Hospital Publisher 1989, 107-112.

2. Sharkis SJ, Santos GW, Colvin OM: Elimination of acute myelogenous leukemic cells from marrow and tumor suspensions in the rat with 4-hydroperoxycyclophosphamide. Blood 1980, 55:521-523.

3. Rowley SC, Jones RJ, Piantadosi S, Braine HG, Colvin OM, Davis J, Saral R, Sharkis S, Wingard J, Yeager AM, Santos GW: Efficacy of ex vivo purging for autologous bone marrow transplantation in the treatment of acute nonlymphoblastic leukemia. Blood 1989, 74:501-506.

4. Gulati SC, Lemoli RM, Acaba L, Igarashi T, Wasserheit C, Mustafa F: Purging in autologous and allogeneic bone marrow transplantation. Current Opinion in Oncology 1992, 4:264-271.

5. Civin CI: Human monomyeloid cell membrane antigens. Exp Hematol 1990, 18:461-467.

6. Ball ED, Mills LE, Coughlin CT, Beck JR, Cornwell GG III: Autologous bone marrow transplantation in acute myelogenous leukemia: In vivo treatment with myeloid cell-specific monoclonal antibodies. Blood 1986, 68:1311-1315.

7. Scheinberg DA, Tanimoto M, McKenzi S, Strife A, Old LJ, Clarkson BD: Monoclonal antibody M195: A diagnostic marker for acute myelogenous leukemia. Leukemia 1989, 3:440-445.

8. Lemoli RM, Gasparetto C, Scheinberg DA, Moore MAS, Clarkson BD, Gulati SC: Autologous bone marrow transplantation in acute myelogenous leukemia: in vitro treatment with myeloid-specific monoclonal antibodies and drugs in combination. Blood 1991, 77:1829-1836.

9. Gross S, Gee AP, Worthington-White DA, eds: Progress in clinical and biological research, bone marrow purging and processing. vol 333 Alan R. Liss Publisher, 1990.

10. Greenberg PL, Baker S, Link M, Minowada J: Immunologic selection of hemopoietic precursor cells utilizing antibody-mediated plate binding ("panning"). Blood 1985, 65:190-197.

11. Pole GJ, Casper J, Elfenbein G, Gee A, Gross S, Jansen W, Koch P, Marcus R, Pick T, Shuster J, Spruce W, Thomas P, Yeager A: High-dose chemo-radiotherapy supported by marrow infusions for advanced neuroblastoma: a Pediatric Oncology Group study. J Clin Oncol 1991, 19:152-158.

12. Shpall EJ, Johnson C, Hami L: Bone marrow purging, In: Armitage JO and Antman HK, ed. High dose cancer therapy. Baltimore, Maryland: Williams and Wilkins Publisher 1992; 249-275.

13. Sutherland DR, Abdullah KM, Cyopick P, Mellors A: Cleavage of the cell-surface O-sialoglycoproteins CD34, CD43, CD44, and CD45 by a novel glyco-protease from Pasteurella haemolytica. J Immunology 1992, 148:1458-1464.

14. Berenson RJ, Bensinger WI, Kalamasz D: Elimination of Daudi lymphoblasts from human bone marrow using avidin-biotin immunoadsorption. Blood 1986, 67:509-515.

15. Berenson RJ, Bensinger WI, Kalamasz D: Positive selection of viable cell populations using avidin-biotin immunoadsorption. J Immunol Methods 1986, 91:11-19.

16. Watt SM, Karhi K, Gatter K, Furley JW, Katz FE, Healy LE, Altan LJ, Bradley NJ, Sutherland DR, Levinsky R, Greaves MF: Distribution and epitope analysis of the cell membrane glycoprotein (HPCA-1) associated with human hematopoietic progenitor cells. Leukemia 1987, 1:417-426.

17. Andrews RG, Bryant EM, Bartelmez SH, Muirhead DY, Knitter GH, Besinger W, Strong DM, Bernstein ID: CD34+ marrow cells, devoid of T and B lymphocytes, reconstitute stable lymphopoiesis and myelopoiesis in lethally irradiated allogeneic baboons. Blood 1992; 80:1693-1701.

18. Shpall EJ, Jones RB, Johnston C, Hami L, Salomon S, Affronti ML, Curiel T, Berenson RJ: Purified CD34 positive marrow progenitor cells provide effective reconstitution for breast cancer and non-Hodgkin's lymphoma patients receiving high dose chemotherapy with autologous bone marrow support: recombinant granulocyte colony stimulating factor accelerates hematopoietic recovery. Proceedings of ASCO 1992; 11:59.

19. Barnett MJ, Eaves CJ, Kalousek DK, Klingermann HG, Lansdorp PM, Reece DE, Shepperd SD, Shaw GH, Eaves AC: Successful autografting in chronic myeloid leukemia after maintenance of marrow in culture. Bone Marrow Transplant 1989, 4:345-351.

20. Cheng J, Morgenstern GR, Coutinho LH, Scarffe JH, Corr T, Deskin DP, Testa NG, Dexter TM: The use of bone marrow cells grown in long-term marrow culture reveals chromosomally normal hematopoietic cells in patients with Philadelphia chromosome-positive chronic myelogenous leukemia: an update. Bone Marrow Transplant 1989 4:5-9.

21. Visani G, Lemoli RM, Dinota A, Galieni P, Gobbi M, Cavo M, Tura S: Evidence that long-term bone marrow culture of patients with multiple myeloma favors normal hemopoietic proliferation. Transplantation 1989, 48:1026-1031.

22. Verfaille C, Blakolner K, McGlave P. Purified primitive human hematopoietic progenitor cells with long-term in vitro repopulating capacity adhere selectively to irradiated bone marrow stroma. J Exp Med 1990, 172:509-520.

23. Coutinho LH, Will A, Radford J, Schiro R, Testa NG, Dexter TM: Effects of recombinant human granulocyte colony-stimulating factor (CSF), human granulocyte-macrophage-CSF and gibbon interleukin-3 on hemopoiesis in human long-term bone marrow culture. Blood 1990, 75:2118-2129.

24. Lemoli RM, Tafuri A, Strife A, Andreeff M, Clarkson BD, Gulati SC:

Proliferation of human hematopoietic progenitors in long-term bone marrow cultures in gas-permeable plastic bags is enhanced by colony-stimulating factors. Exp Hematol 1992, 20:569-575.

25. Schneider JG, Crown J, Shapiro F, Reich L, Hoskins I, Hakes T, Norton L, Moore MAS: Ex vivo cytokine expansion of CD34-positive hemato-poietic progenitors in bone marrow, placental cord blood, and cyclophos-phamide & G-CSF mobilized peripheral blood. Blood 1992; 80(Suppl 1):268a.

26. Gimble JM, Medina K, Hudson J, Robinson M, Kincade PW: Modula-tion of lymphohematopoiesis in long-term culturs by gamma interferon: direct and indirect action on lymphoid and stromal cells. Exp Hematol-ogy 1993; 21:224-230.

27. Moore MAS: Does stem cell exhaustion result from combining hemato-poietic growth factors with chemotherapy? If so, how do we prevent it? Blood 1992; 80:3-7.

28. Yau JC, Reading CL, Thomas MW, Davaraj BM, Tindle SE, Jagannath S, Dicke KA: Purging of T-lymphocytes with magnetic affinity colloid. Exp Hematol 1990, 18:219-222.

29. Filipovich AH, Youle RJ, Neville DM, Vallera DA, Quinones RR, Kersey JH: Ex vivo treatment of donor bone marrow and anti-T-cell immunotoxins for prevention of graft-versus-host disease. Lancet 1984, i:469-472.

30. Soiffer RJ, Murray C, Mauch P, Anderson KC, Freedman AS, Rabinowe SN, Takvorian T, Robertson MJ, Spector N, Gonin R, Miller KB, Rudders RA, Freeman A, Blake K, Coral F, Nadler LM, Ritz J: Prevention of graft-versus-host disease by selective depletion of CD6-positive T-lymphocytes from donor bone marrow. J of Clinl Oncol 1992; 10:1191-1200.

31. Siena S, Castro-Malaspina H, Gulati SC, Lu L, Colvin MO, Clarkson BD, O'Reilly RJ, Moore MAS: Effects of in vitro purging with 4-hydroperoxycyclophosphamide on the hematopoietic and microenvi-ronmental elements of human bone marrow. Blood 1985, 65:655-662.

32. Jones RJ: Purging with 4-hydroperoxycyclophosphamide. J of Hematotherapy, 1992, 1:343-348.

33. Gulati SC, Atzpodien J, Langleben A, Shimazaki C, Jain Kirti, Yopp J, Ng RP, Colvin OM, Clarkson BD: Comparative regimens for the ex vivo chemopurification of B cell lymphoma-contaminated marrow. Act Haematologica 1988, 80:65-70.

34. Atzpodien J, Gulati SC, Clarkson BD: Comparison of the Cytotoxic effects of merocyanine-540 on leukemic cells and normal human bone marrow. Cancer Research 1986, 46:4892-4895.

35. Chou T-C, Talalay P: Quantitative analysis of dose-effects relationships: the combined effect of multiple drugs on enzyme inhibitors. Adv Enzyme Regul 1985; 22:27-55.

36. Chang T-T, Gulati SC, Chou T-C, Colvin M, Clarkson BD: Compara-tive cytotoxicity of various drug combinations for human leukemic cells and normal hematopoietic precursors. Cancer Research 1987; 47:119-122.

37. Hilton J: Role of aldehyde dehydrogenase in cyclophosphamide-resistant L1210 leukemia. Cancer Res 1984, 44:5156-5160.

38. Cardoso AA, Fallon M, Mukherji Bijay, Silva MR, Marusic M, Gaffney J, Ascensao JL: Effect of pharmacological purging on natural killer cell number and activity in human bone marrow. Clin Immunol and Immunopathology 1992, 64:106-111.

39. Kushner BH, Kwon JH, Gulati SC, Castro-Malaspina H: Preclinical assessment of purging with VP-16-213: key role for long-term marrow cultures. Blood 1987, 69:65-71.

40. Lemoli RM, Gulati SC: In vitro cytotoxicity of VP-16-213 and nitrogen mustard: Agonistic on tumor cells but not on normal human bone marrow progenitors. Exp Hematol 1990, 18:1008-1012.

41. Stiff PJ, Schulz WC, Bishop M, Marks L: Anti-CD33 monoclonal antibody and etoposide/cytosine arabinoside combinations for the ex vivo purification of bone marrow in acute nonlymphocytic leukemia. Blood 1991, 77:355-362.

42. Atzpodien J, Wisniewski D, Gulati S, Welte K, Knowles R, Clarkson B: Interleukin-2 and mitogen-activated NK-like killer cells from highly purified human peripheral blood T-cell (CD3+ N901-). Nat Immun Growth Regul 1987; 6:129-140.

43. Takaue Y, Roome AJ, Turpin JA, Reading CL: Depletion of T-lymphocytes from human bone marrow by the use of counterflow elutriation centrifugation. Am J Hematol 1986, 23:247-262.

44. Pierelli L, Menichella G, Serafini R, de Martini M, Paoloni A, Foddai ML, Scambia G, Benedetti Panici PL, Mancuso S, Leone G, Mango G, Bizzi B: Autologous bone marrow processing for autotransplantation using an automated cell processor and a semiautomated procedure. Bone Marrow Transplantation 1991;7:355-361.

45. Glasser L, Fiederlein RL, Dalton WA, Vogler WR: The effect of alkyl-lysophospholipids (ALP) on human myeloma cell lines. Blood 1992, 80 (Suppl 1):484.

46. Vogler W, Berdel W, Olson A, Winton E, Heffner L, Gordon D: Autologous bone marrow transplantation in acute leukemia with marrow purged with alkyl-lysophospholipid. Blood 1992; 80:1423-1429.

47. Sieber F, Spivak JL, Sutcliffe AM: Selective killing of leukemic cells by merocyanine 540-mediated photosensitization. Proc Natl Acad Sci USA 1984, 81:7584-7587.

48. Atzpodien J, Gulati SC, Clarkson BC: Photoradiation models for the clinical ex vivo treatment of autologous bone marrow grafts. Blood 1987, 70:484-489.

49. Gulati SC, Atzpodien J, Lemoli R, Shimazaki S, Clarkson BD: Photoradiation methods for purging autologous bone marrow grafts. Progress Clin Biol Res 1990; 333:87-102.

50. Lemoli RM, Igarashi T, Knizewski M, Acaba L, Richter A, Jain A, Mitchell D, Levy J, Gulati SC: Dye-mediated photolysis is capable of eliminating drug-resistant tumor cells. Blood 1993; 31:793-800.

51. Evensen JF, Sommer S, Moan J, Christensen T: Tumor-localizing and photosensitizing properties of the main components of hematoporphyrin derivative. Cancer Res 1984; 44:482-486.

52. Lotem J, Sachs L: Hematopoietic cytokines inhibit apoptosis induced by transforming growth factor B1 and cancer chemotherapy compounds in myeloid leukemic cells. Blood 1992; 80:1750-1757.

53. Hauch M, Gazzola MV, Small T, Bordignon C, Barnett L, Cunningham I, Castro-Malaspina H, O'Reilly RJ, Keever CA: Anti-leukemia potential of interleukin-2 activated natural killer cells after bone marrow transplantation for chronic myelogenous leukemia. Blood 1990; 75:2250-2262.

54. Gulati SC, Shimazaki C, Lemoli RM, Atzpodien J, Clarkson BD: Ex vivo treatment of myeloma cells by 4-HC, VP-16, LAK cells and antibodies. Eur J Haematol 1989; 43(Suppl 51):164-172.

55. Chleq-Deschamps CM, LeBrun DP, Huie P, Besnier DP, Warnke RA, Sibley RK, Cleary ML: Topographical dissociation of BCL-2 messenger RNA and protein expression in human lymphoid tissues. Blood 1993; 81:293-298.

56. Vaux DL, Weissman IL, Kim SK: Prevention of programmed cell death in caenorhabditis elegans by human bcl-2. Science 1992; 258:1955-1957.

57. Szczylik C, Skorski T, Nicolaides NC, Manzella L, Malaguarnera L, Donatella V, Gewirtz AM, Calabretta B: Selective inhibition of leukemia cell proliferation by BCR-ABL antisense oligodeoxynucleotides. Science 1991; 253:562-565.

58. Uckun FM, Kersey JH, Vallera DA, Ledbetter JA, Weisorf D, Myers DE, Haake R, Ramsay KC: Autologous bone marrow transplantation in high risk remission T-lineage acute lymphoblastic leukemia using immunotoxins plus 4-HC for marrow purging. Blood 1990; 1723-1733.

59. Aihara M, Sikic BI, Blume KG, Chao NJ: Assessment of purging with multidrug resistance (MDR) modulators and VP-16: results of long-term marrow culture. Exp Hematol 1990; 18:940-944.

60. Smoluk GD, Fahey RC: Radioprotection of cells in culture by WR-2721 and derivatives: form of the drug responsible for protection. Cancer Res 1988; 48:3641-3647.

CHAPTER 3

STORAGE AND CRYOPRESERVATION OF STEM CELLS

Improvements in cryopreservation of biological material has been ongoing for the last several years. Cryopreservation of sperm is now routinely performed especially prior to treatment of young male patients with cancer. Cryoprotectants usually work by decreasing the ice crystal formation when liquid water goes through the transition phase into the solid ice state.[1-8] Cells can also be injured by the direct effects of low temperatures. Intracellular ice formation occurring with high rates of cooling may rupture the cell. Extracellular ice formation results in progressive increase in the osmolality of the extracellular medium as water is taken up by the growing ice crystals, resulting in severe dehydration of the cell. Macromolecular cryoprotectants such as hydroxyethyl starch (HES) remain external to the cell and appear to provide protection by undergoing a reversible "glass transition", forming a viscous shell around the cell and thereby preventing water shifts and progressive cellular dehydration.[6] Penetrating cryoprotectants such as dimethylsulfoxide (DMSO) and glycerol afford protection by their colligative properties and lower the freezing temperature of the medium, thus reducing the proportion of water incorporated into ice and the extent of cellular dehydration. For a compound to be a colligative cryoprotectant, it must be capable of permeating the cell otherwise it would merely add to the extracellular osmolality. It must also be nontoxic to the cells. Stem cells are usually not cryopreserved in glycerol, because glycerol can cause lactic acidosis when infused into the patient. Washing out glycerol from the stem cells is a cumbersome process and often results in loss of cell viability.

DMSO has been the primary cryoprotectant used by most autologous marrow transplant programs because it has minor toxicity upon infusion into the patient. DMSO is also relatively permeable across the cell membrane, and the thawed cell suspension need not be washed or diluted before reinfusion. However, DMSO is not without toxicity. Reports of cardiac dysfunction, anaphylaxis, and a variety of somatic complaints have been associated with the reinfusion of cryopreserved stem cells.[8-11]

A direct chemical toxicity of DMSO to hematopoietic progenitors has been suggested.[12,13] Both short-term and prolonged exposures to this compound have been reported to cause loss of hematopoietic progenitors. Thus, minimizing exposure times of cells to DMSO before freezing, and developing cryoprotectant solutions containing reduced DMSO concentrations were evaluated. In one recent study,[14] chemical toxicity of DMSO to myeloid and erythroid progenitor cells from healthy donors was evaluated. No DMSO toxicity was found in concentrations of 5% or 10% at either 4°C or 37°C for incubation durations up to 1 hour. DMSO at 20% did not decrease the number of progenitor cell-derived colonies per $5x10^4$ cells cultured, but did induce cell clumping during DMSO washout, resulting in a net loss of progenitor cells. At a concentration of 40% DMSO, a direct toxicity to hematopoietic progenitors was found. Delay in removal of DMSO after thawing of cryopreserved cells for periods up to 1 hour was also not toxic to hematopoietic progenitor cells. Direct addition of DMSO at 1% or 10% final concentration (v/v) to the culture dishes suppressed colony formation. These data suggest that DMSO may not be toxic to hematopoietic progenitor cells after short-term exposure at the concentrations used for cryopreservation of marrow and peripheral blood stem cells.[14] Investigations at Memorial Sloan-Kettering Cancer Center revealed that a mixture of 5% DMSO, 4% albumin, and 6% HES is very effective in cryopreserving platelets and hematopoietic stem cells.[15-17] These methods are being used without controlled rate freezing.

Several authors believe that leukemic cells do not cryopreserve as well as normal hematopoietic cells.[18-19] In one study,[18] six different freezing conditions were utilized and all of the freezing mixtures tested were ineffective in preserving leukemic cells. Approximately 1% of the leukemic cells were found to be viable after cryopreservation. Stem cells cryopreserved in DMSO may demonstrate a decrease in the proliferation of malignant cells, because DMSO can promote differentiation resulting in loss of proliferative and malignant potential. Effect of DMSO on the differentiation of leukemic cells is well-known.

Various machines can be used for cryopreservation. Approximately 70% of the centers utilize control rate freezing apparatus and then store the cells in vapor or liquid phase of nitrogen. Newer generation of electrical freezers can achieve temperatures of -135°C and are being used without a separate control rate freezing apparatus with increasing frequency. Figure 1 describes

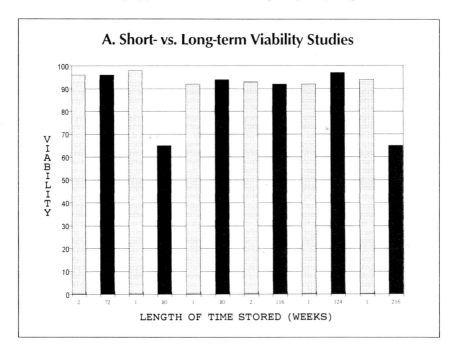

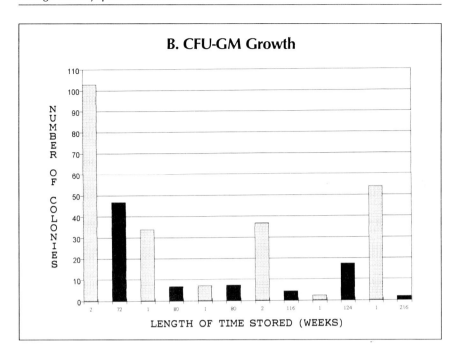

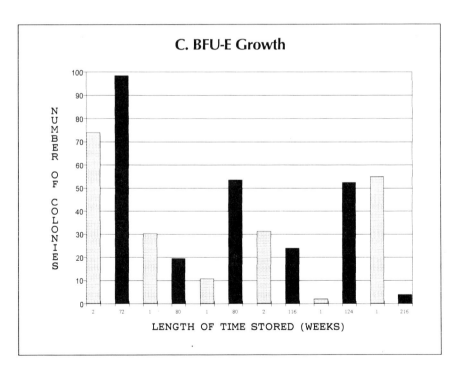

Figure 1. Cells cryopreserved at -110 to -135°C were thawed and evaluated for viability (A); colony forming units - granulocyte, macrophage (CFU-GM) (B); and erythroid burst forming units (BFU-e) (C). The analysis was performed after 1-2 weeks (short-term storage, dotted bars) or after 72-216 weeks (long-term storage, solid bars).

Table 1. Difference in storage at -120°C vs -196°C

VIABILITY AFTER FREEZE THAWING		
	-120°C	-196°C
1-2 months	91% (87-94)[3]	84% (84-90)[3]
3 months	89.5% (89-90)[2]	89.5% (88-91)[2]
7 months	90% [1]	90% [1]
[# of patients]		

the quality of bone marrow cryopreservation in electric freezers. The data of bone marrow cells frozen at -196°C and at -120°C are compared in Table 1. In one patient, acceptable hematopoietic engraftment was obtained with BM cryopreserved for 216 weeks. All hematopoietic lineages were present 18 days after transplantation. Subsequently, the patient died of acute respiratory distress syndrome.

In a recent publication, the clinical toxicity of cryopreserved bone marrow infusion in 82 patients was reported.[8] All BM were cryopreserved in 10% DMSO and stored in liquid nitrogen. Varying symptoms of nausea, abdominal cramping, and flushing were noted. Forced vital capacity of the lungs decreased in most patients receiving concentrated cells. A significant group of patients developed transient hypertension, with 38% of these patients requiring additional medications within six hours. In one series,[20] the risk of bacterial contamination was reported to be 17% but usually bacterial contamination is not a problem in modern day laboratories with the use of aseptic techniques. One interesting approach is to store stem cells for short periods in refrigerator (up to 56 hours), patient undergoes cytotoxic therapy (utilize drugs with short half life) and then reinfuse the cells stored at 4°C.[21] It is of interest that refrigerated marrow has faster recovery of platelet count. Such approaches should be used with appropriate training, preclinical evaluation and with attention to quality controls. Most likely, cryopreserved stem cells are biologically active for 2-4 years. Reliable assays which predict the biological function of cryopreserved stem cells and guidelines to decide how long to keep cells frozen need to be developed. Bone marrow harvest can now be performed on an out-patient basis.[22] Appropriate management of purged cells prior to reinfusion into the patient is an important aspect of autologous stem cell transplantation and should be performed with care.

REFERENCES

1. Polge C. Smith AU, Parkes AS: Revival of spermatozoa after vitrification and dehydration at low temperatures. Nature 1949; 164:666.
2. Mazur P, Cole KW, Hall JW, Schreuders PD, Mahowald AP: Cryobiological Preservation of Drosophila Embryos. Science 1992; 258:1932-1935.
3. Lovelock JE, Bishop MWH: Prevention of freezing damage to living cells

by dimethylsulfoxide. Nature 1959; 183:1394.

4. Ashwood-Smith MJ, Warby C, Connor KW: Low temperature preservation of mammalian cells in tissue culture with polyvinylpyrrolidone (PVP), dextrans, hydroxyethylstarch (HES). Cryobiology 1972; 9:441.

5. Karow AM, Webb WR. Tissue freezing. A theory for injury and survival. Cryobiology 1965; 2:99-108.

6. Takahashi T, Hirsh A, Erbe E, Williams RJ. Mechanism of cryoprotection by extracellular polymeric solutes. Biophy J 1988; 54:509-518.

7. Mazur P. Fundamental cryobiology and the preservation of organs by freezing. In: Karow AM, Pegg DE, eds. Organ preservation for transplantation. Marcel Dekker, Inc., New York, 1981; 143-175.

8. Davis JM, Rowley SD, Braine HG,Piantadosi, Santos GW. Clinical toxicity of cryopreserved bone marrow graft infusion. Blood 1990; 75:781-786.

9. Rapoport AP, Rowe JM, Packman CH, Ginsberg SJ. Cardiac arrest after autologous marrow infusion. Bone Marrow Transplantation 1991; 7:401-403.

10. Kessinger A, Schmit-Pokorny K, Smith D, Armitage J. Cryopreservation and infusion of autologous peripheral blood stem cells. Bone Marrow Transplantation 1990; 5 (suppl 1):25-27.

11. Stroncek DF, Fautsch SK, Lasky LC, Hurd DD, Ramsay NKC, McCullough J. Adverse reactions in patients transfused with cryopreserved marrow. Transfusion 1991; 31:521-526.

12. Douay L, Gorin NC, David R, Stachowiak J, Salmon C, Najman A, Duhamel G. Study of granulocyte-macrophage progenitor (CFU$_c$) preservation after slow freezing of bone marrow in the gas phase of liquid nitrogen. Experimental Hematology 1982; 10:360-366.

13. Goldman JM, Th'ng KH, Park DS, Spiers AS, Lowenthal RM, Ruutu T. Collection, cryopreservation and subsequent viability of haemopoietic stem cells intended for treatment of chronic granulocytic leukaemia in blast-cell transformation. Brit J Haematol 1978; 40:185-195.

14. Rowley SC, Anderson GL. Effect of dimethylsulfoxide exposure without cryopreservation on hematopoietic progenitor cells. BMT 1993 (accepted).

15. Zaroulis CF, Liederman I: Successful freeze-preservation of human granulocytes. Cryobiology 1980; 17:311-317.

16. Stiff PJ, DeRisi MF, Langleben A, Gulati SC, Koester A, Lanzotti V, Clarkson B: Autologous bone marrow transplantation using unfractionated cells without rate-controlled freezing in hydroxyethyl starch and dimethyl sulfoxide. Ann NY Acad Sci 1983; 411:378-380.

17. Stiff PJ, Koester AR, Weidner MK, Dvorak K, Fisher RI: Autologous bone marrow transplantation using unfractionated cells cryopreserved in dimethylsulfoxide and hydroxyethyl starch without controlled-rate freezing. Blood 1987; 70:974-979.

18. Allieri MA, Lopez M, Douay, Martini E, Deloux H, Giarratana C, Najman A, Gorin NC: Intrinsic leukemic progenitor cells sensitivity to cryopreservation: incidence for autologous bone marrow transplantation. In Dicke KA, Spitzer G, Jagannath S (eds). Autologous Bone Marrow Transplantation: Proc Fourth Intl Symp 1988; MD Anderson Hospital Publishers, Houston, 3:35-39.

19. Bouroncle BA. Preservation of human normal and leukemic cells with dimethyl sulfoxide at -80°C. Cryobiology 1967; 3:445-455.

20. Rowley SD, Davis J, Dick DJ, Briane HG, Charache P, Saral R, Sensenbrenner LL, Santos GW: Bacterial contamination of bone marrow grafts intended for autologous and allogeneic bone marrow transplantation; incidence and clinical significance. Transfusion 1988; 28:109-112.

21. Carey P, Proctor SJ, Taylor P, Hamilton PJ: Autologous bone marrow transplantation for high grade lymphoid malignancy using Melphalan/ irradiation conditioning without marrow purging or cryopreservation. Blood 1991; 77:1593-1598.

22. Thorne AC, Stewart M, Gulati SC: Harvesting bone marrow in an out-patient setting using newer anesthetic agents. 1993; JCO 11: 320-323.

CHAPTER 4

RESULTS OF PURGING IN HEMATOLOGICAL MALIGNANCIES

The success of autologous stem cell transplantation (AUSCT) depends on the availability of normal hematopoietic elements to engraft the patient after hematoablative therapy. Hematological malignancies usually coexist with and/or even effect the early hematopoietic precursors and may therefore have marked reduction or absence of normal hematopoietic precursors. The current knowledge of various mechanisms that may be involved in hematological malignancies are briefly updated below. A better understanding of the molecular changes in hematological malignancies will help in deciding which patients will benefit from AUSCT and will aid in deciding the best conditioning and BM purging regimens.[1-7]

The complex hematopoietic system probably arises from a small number of stem cells that during embryogenesis may replenish, differentiate and migrate into various organs in the fetal tissue. As embryogenesis progresses, the hematopoietic compartment moves into the bone marrow. The true hematopoietic stem cell may exist only in early stages of embryogenesis, but in adults one or a small number of hematopoietic cells may be able to sustain the hematopoietic growth. These stem cells are able to self-replicate and differentiate into various lineages. The differentiated hematopoietic elements gradually lose the self-renewal capacity, and recent work has elegantly shown that irreversible changes occur in DNA during differentiation. The alterations in genetic material have been defined for lymphoid cells.[5-7]

Various growth factors and cells of different lineages (especially T-lymphocytes and activated macrophages) either directly or indirectly (through growth factors) control the quality and quantity of different hematopoietic subgroups so that an orderly balance of each cell population is maintained. Any abnormality in such regulation may result in preferential growth advantage for one lineage over the other and probably accounts for the neoplastic growth. Various factors may trigger these mechanisms of neoplastic growth.[4-10]

ACUTE MYELOBLASTIC LEUKEMIA

Various cytogenetic defects are found in patients with acute non-lymphoblastic leukemia, and patients are now often subgrouped by cytogenetic defect for prognosis. Most authors subgroup patients with t(8,12); inv, t(16,16); t(9,11); 11q abnormality and t(15,17) as having good prognosis and patients with inv 3, +3; -7/7q - and -5/5q changes as having poor prognosis.[11] The above changes imply damage at different locations and probably affect various stages of differentiation, that is, t(15,17) abnormality is noted in patients with acute promyelocytic leukemia (APL, M_3 by FAB classification) and probably contributes to the hypergranular myeloid cells in this disease.[12] Clearly, the unique response to trans-retinoic acid may have an interaction with the gene/gene product(s) of this chromosomal abnormality. Attempts have also been made to correlate various oncogene expressions (N-myc, C-myb, C-fes, etc.) and overall prognoses in different types of leukemia and other cancers. Biphenotypic leukemia is another example where the defect is probably in the earlier precursor stage of the two lineages involved, and the lymphoid and myeloid series are often involved.

With the advent of newer combination chemotherapies, 60% to 80% of patients with acute myelogenous leukemia (AML) can now achieve remission. Most protocols combine continuous infusion of cytosine arabinoside (Ara-C) with an anthracycline. Despite modifications in the dose and scheduling of these drugs, most patients relapse; and long-term survival rarely exceeds 15%-35%.[13-15] Various consolidation and maintenance sequences have not substantially improved the overall survival, except for patients with APL in first remission, and the need for various post-remission therapies is difficult to demonstrate because of concomitant improvement in the overall management of patients with leukemia.

BMT

Considering the possibility of relapse occurring from minimal residual disease after remission is attained, various centers have utilized hematoablative dosages of drugs known to be effective against leukemic cells. Hematopoietic reconstitution can then be obtained by using allogeneic bone marrow transplantation (ALBMT) or autologous stem cell transplantation (using BM or peripheral blood stem cells) AUSCT. Patients undergoing ALBMT may do slightly better than patients receiving consolidation therapy.[16,17] Encouraging clinical results have been reported with AUSCT. Some centers have utilized bone marrow obtained in remission, frozen without any additional treatment (nonpurged) but most centers utilize various methods to purge the bone marrow of any residual leukemic cells. The methods and dosage utilized for purging bone marrow are usually different in the studies reported. 4-Hydroperoxycyclophosphamide (4-HC, the active metabolite of cyclophosphamide) and its analogues were the first agents used in purging the bone marrow of patients with AML.[18,19] VP-16 alone is also a useful drug for purging leukemic cells. At MSKCC, the patient's BM is purged with a combination of 4-HC and VP-16. The patient's conditioning regimen consists of total body irradiation 1,320 rads delivered over 4 days in 11 (eleven) fractions, VP-16 250 mg/m² IV per day for 3 days and cyclophosphamide 60 mg/kg/day IV for 2 days. The results are described in Figure 1.[20] In vitro treatment of bone marrow with VP-16 and 4-HC resulted in 86% median inhibition of colony-forming units-granulocyte macrophage (CFU-GM) and 83% median inhibition of burst-forming units-erythroid (BFU-E) in the assay of the infused bone marrow. Despite this marked inhibition in hematopoietic progenitors, all patients had hematopoietic recovery. The platelet counts of one patient failed to reach 50,000/mcL and he subsequently relapsed. The median number of days to achieve a white blood cell (WBC) count of greater than 1,000/mcL, a neutrophil count of greater than 500/mcL and an unsupported platelet count of 50,000/mcL was 32 (range 13 to 53) days, 32 (range 21 to 53) days, and 64 (range 15 to 279) days respectively. None of the variables of the purging procedure (the cell dose administered, the concentration of VP-16, the % viability of the infused bone marrow, the inhibition of CFU-GM and BFU-E in the treated marrow) were associated with the rate of hematological reconstitution in this small study sample.[20]

The need for in vitro treatment of autografts has been questioned. In a recent analysis of 1,483 patients with AML from the European Bone Marrow Transplant Study group, the data was analyzed to evaluate the benefit of AUBMT over long follow-up time (maximum of over 11 years) and also to understand the influence of pre-transplant interval, purging, etc. It was confirmed that longer intervals from remission to AUBMT were associated with better leukemia-free survival (LFS) and lower relapse rate in AML.[19] The cut-off was three months in CR1 and six months in CR2. Two factors could explain these findings: first, a selection bias, since patients transplanted late being already at a lower risk of relapse when AUBMT was performed; second, a potential beneficial effect from additional consolidation courses which would reduce the residual tumor load in the marrow collected (in vivo

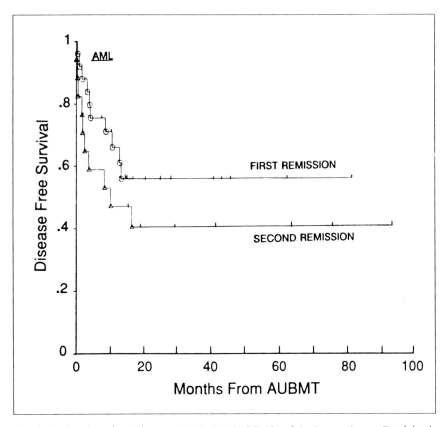

Figure 1. Results of autologous BMT at MSKCC. Conditioning regimen: Total body irradiation, VP-16 and cyclophosphamide. Bone marrow purged with 4-HC and VP-16.

purging). Several studies have demonstrated that patients reaching CR1 more rapidly have the best prognosis. The introduction of AUBMT in the therapeutic strategy treatment did not modify the influence of this factor. Patients reaching CR1 within 40 days had a better LFS than those reaching CR later (51 versus 35%). It was also found that the prognosis of patients transplanted in CR2 was related to the duration of CR1, with better LFS in those with longest CR1 duration. Similar observations were noted in MRC AML 9 trial. This study also confirmed the previous observation that purging efficacy in AML CR1 was easier to detect and/or more important in the subgroup of patients where the probability of persistance of residual tumor was higher, i.e., patients transplanted earlier post CR (≤6 months) and slow remitters following initial induction (>40 days).[19]

Several institutions are utilizing peripheral blood stem cell transplantation (PBSCT) for patients with AML.[21,22] The use of PBSC as opposed to bone marrow cells may be associated with two advantages. Firstly, several pilot studies indicate that the speed of engraftment following autologous PBSCT is similar to or better than that observed after autologous bone marrow transplantation (AUBMT). Secondly, it has been hypothesized that PBSC may be less contaminated by residual leukemic cells than bone marrow cells, and that the risk of relapse following PBSCT may be less than that observed after AUBMT. So far, no significant difference in survival has been noted when PBSCT (unpurged) are used when compared to purged AUBMT. Improvements in the use of both technologies and proper monitoring to compare differences in the relapse rate (and other toxicities) will help decide which therapy is better after long-term analysis. Unfortunately, most investigators are not involved in proper scientific studies in this regard.

Further studies will be needed to determine the efficacy of purging in 2nd R or 3rd R and optimal purging agents. Novel purging methods may be needed for complete eradication of occult viable leukemic cells. Recently, chemo-immunopurging with VP-16/Ara-C followed by complement mediated lysis using a myeloid monoclonal antibody (anti-CD33) in vitro has been shown to synergistically kill clonogenic leukemic cells while sparing early hematopoietic progenitor cells.[23]

Some investigators are pursuing selective T-cell purged allogeneic BMT with the intent of exploiting the graft-versus-leukemia effect seen in patients who develop grade I-II graft-versus-host disease (GVHD). The ALBMT benefit is mainly restricted to younger patients as the incidence of side effects, especially GVHD and graft failure is higher in older patients.[16,17] It has been suggested that patients with GVHD may have a lower leukemic relapse rate after ALBMT due to graft-versus-leukemic affect.[16,17] Various methods to deplete the graft bone marrow of T-lymphocytes have shown a decrease in GVHD and its related morbidity.[18] However, there has been an interesting observation that the incidence of graft failures is especially high with male donors when the bone marrow is depleted of lymphocytes using soybean-lectin separation methods.[18] Various methods are now being evaluated to decrease the rate of graft rejection. Overall, the results of ALBMT in first remission (1st R) are better than those of ALBMT in 1st early relapse or second remission (2nd R). The results of ALBMT in florid relapse are even worse.[16,17] Several institutions are comparing conventional post-remission chemotherapy with allogeneic and autologous BMT in 1st remission in randomized clinical trials.

In one randomized study, 116 adult patients aged 14-73 with previously untreated acute myeloid leukemia received induction and consolidation chemotherapy with daunorubicin, cytosine arabinoside and thioguanine. Two novel approaches to post-consolidation therapy were investigated. Patients aged 50 years or less who had no suitable matched allogeneic donor were considered for autologous bone marrow transplantation (BMT), using bone marrow purged by 14-day culture in vitro. Patients over the age of 50 years with normal bone marrow cellularity and peripheral blood count were treated with a single oral dose of busulphan 100 mg/m^2 (without BMT rescue) three months following the completion of consolidation therapy. Eighty-seven patients (75%) achieved a complete remission. Of 70 patients who completed consolidation therapy, 40 were aged $\leq$ 50 years and 30 were > 50 years. Forty-three patients went on to receive post consolidation therapy in first CR (autologous BMT 12, allogeneic BMT 7, busulphan therapy 24). The event-free survival at 4 years was 47% for autologous BMT, 34% for allogeneic BMT and 45% for busulphan-treated patients. The survival for the older cohort of patients who received post-consolidation therapy with single dose busulphan therapy was encouraging, and suggests that improved post-consolidation therapy even without BMT (allogeneic or autologous) may be useful in treating patients with AML.[24]

A significant portion of the patients are unable to undergo transplantation, even after proper initial therapy because of various medical reasons.[14] Most often the disease progresses. Showing concern about the development of drug resistance to initial therapy (use of verapamil, cyclosporine, etc. upfront with initial therapy), and perhaps using alternating therapies for induction and consolidation will increase the number of patients suitable for transplantation. This may decrease the time before patients qualify for AUBMT or ALBMT and thus decrease the variability in response noted in the current literature.

The role of ALBMT, AUBMT or intensive chemotherapy in patients with AML who achieve remission is controversial. Although the definition of complete remission implies prognostic significance for patients with lymphoma, unfortunately in patients with AML, minimal residual leukemia is difficult to diagnose and except in a rare situation where cytogenetics and polymerase chain reaction (PCR) technology is useful, it is difficult to determine which patient will relapse. Obtaining remission (less than 5% blasts) is very important in overall prognosis of patients with AML. The results of ALBMT are probably equivalent or slightly superior to those attained with intensive chemotherapy. This is especially true for older patients and the long-term survival ranges from 20% to 40% after ALBMT and chemotherapy. Fifty to sixty percent DFS reported in 1st remission with AUBMT compares favorably to ALBMT and intensive chemotherapy. Higher relapse rates reported in some series with AUBMT may be due to the loss of the graft-versus-leukemia effect, which may be of some benefit to patients undergoing ALBMT.

In patients with AML in second or third R there is less controversy regarding therapy, since intensive chemotherapy results in few cures with a long-term survival of only 5%. The results of ALBMT in first relapse or early second are nearly equivalent to AUBMT results reporting 30-40% DFS. The mortality of AUBMT is slightly lower than ALBMT where late deaths occur (usually due to GVHD).

Unresponsive disease (primary resistance and relapse) remains the main problem for patients with AML and unfortunately, in a significant number of patients relapse occurs due to the development of drug resistance, not only to the anthracycline but also to Ara-C. Considering that the usual initial therapy of AML revolves around various doses and schedules of Ara-C and an anthracycline, various less active but still reasonably effective drugs, such as vincristine, CTX, or VP-16, immunomodulation methods, or drugs to decrease the development of resistance should be evaluated up-front. Some of these concepts are presently being evaluated in clinical trials. Future trials should explore the role of new innovative approaches to decrease the relapse rate and toxicity of the treatment for patients with AML.

ACUTE LYMPHOBLASTIC LEUKEMIA

Acute lymphoblastic leukemia (ALL) is a common leukemia in children. In adults, approximately 20% of the patients are diagnosed to have ALL. During the last two decades, progress has been made in the identification of prognostic factors helping to define low and high risk patients and in the development of intensified treatment strategies.[25-38] In adults, long-term remission rates of 20-35% have been reported for patients with ALL and lymphoblastic lymphoma.[25] The success is primarily due to the improvement of induction therapy and early consolidation. Nevertheless, more than 50% of the patients who attain a complete remission will relapse, and most salvage regimens, with the possible exception of allogeneic bone marrow transplantation (ALBMT), are ineffective.[28,33,34] Recent advances in understanding the heterogenic pathobiology of adult ALL, especially the cytogenetic diversity, have provided new diagnostic methods and valuable prognostic information. The development of alternative and more aggressive treatment protocols, including escalating doses of cytotoxic drugs, bone marrow transplantation, use of growth factors, and various biological response modifiers, requires further investigation. Treatment designs will also have to concentrate on improved strategies to decrease the development of drug resistance in the leukemic cell.

PATHOPHYSIOLOGY

ALL is a neoplastic disease with clonal expansion of immature lymphoblastic cells. The morphological classification of ALL by the FAB Cooperative Study Group (L1-L3) has been extended by the application of monoclonal antibodies for immunophenotyping and improved cytogenetic evaluation of neoplastic lymphoblasts. This classification of ALL includes (1) early precursor B-cell ALL, (2) common ALL, (3) pre-B-ALL, (4) B-cell-ALL; and (1) early-T-precursor ALL and (2) T-cell ALL for T-cell derived neoplasia. Several findings focus on the concept of viral leukemogenesis for some patients with ALL.[29] HTLV-1 genomic sequences have been identified in adult T-cell leukemia/lymphoma (ATL) cells. These malignancies are clustered geographically in Japan, the Caribbean and certain parts of Africa and America, suggesting etiological relevance of infectious agents. The genome of the trans-activating retrovirus HTLV-1 encodes for the p40 tax protein, that has been found to be associated with the transcriptional activation of cytokine genes, such as the IL-2, IL-6, IL-9, GM-CSF, IL-2 receptor α chain (tac), and

TGF-beta 1 genes and the c-fos oncogene.[29,35] These findings would suggest that in some patients, especially with T-cell ALL, purging methods may have to be different or may fail because of genomic involvement of the entire hematopoietic lineage.

Clonal abnormalities of chromosomes, affecting either their number (hyperdiploid, hypodiploid, pseudodiploid) or structure, are frequent findings in adult ALL (approximately 25%) and have been shown to be predictive of patient's outcome. Some of these structural aberrations are associated with the activation of proto-oncogenes. The most frequent structural abnormality in adult ALL patients is the translocation t(9;22). Bcr-abl rearrangements are detected in up to 43% of patients over 50 years old and are associated with a poor prognosis.[28,30] Other nonrandom translocations are the t(8;14), first described in Burkitt lymphoma, with activation of the c-myc oncogene, and the t(4;11), which is usually associated with a higher frequency of biphenotypic leukemic cells. Experiments designed to study the involvement of other oncogenes in adult ALL do not provide consistent data. Especially in adult ALL, the high degree of genomic diversity and the loss of karyotypic stability has to be considered. Alterations of the p53 tumor suppressor gene resulting in loss-off-function mutations with neoplastic potential were demonstrated in adult T-cell leukemia. Other trials confirm increased p53 mutations in Burkitt lymphoma and L3 ALL.[31]

TREATMENT

Conventional cytotoxic drugs in ALL remission induction therapy are vincristine and prednisone, often combined with an anthracycline (daunorubicin, doxorubicin) and L-asparaginase. Complete remission rates of 75% to 94% have been reported with these regimens. High-dose chemotherapy for remission induction has not substantially improved remission rates. Optimal post-remission therapy in adult ALL remains to be determined. Multidrug treatment protocols for intensification, consolidation, and maintenance therapy were associated with complete remission rates of about 80% and five-year probability of survival is estimated to be at 35-45%.[25-28]

The high-risk group of patients with ALL have been successfully treated with matched sibling marrow transplantation, resulting in 25 to 60% of patients cured, depending on the risk group transplanted. For patients who lack a histocompatible donor, studies initiated in Minneapolis and Boston demonstrated that patients without a sibling donor can be successfully transplanted with autologous purged marrow and that about 20% of these patients were projected to be long-term disease-free survivors.[36] An analysis of patients transplanted at the University of Minnesota to the end of 1992 compared results in high risk ALL in patients who received the various donor types. Follow-up of 44 related donor transplants projects a 29% disease-free survival. A total of 17 patients with high risk ALL were transplanted using an unrelated donor with a projected disease-free survival of 28%.[37] Follow-up of 105 autologous transplants projects a 9% disease free survival. Thus, in these analyses, the results of autologous marrow transplantation appear inferior to those of matched sibling or unrelated transplants. The primary cause of failure is leukemic relapse in all groups. However, nonrelapse mortality accounts for a significant number of failures in the related and matched sibling donors while relapses account for almost all the failures in the group who receive autologous grafts. The considerable biological heterogeneity of adult ALL suggests that we may have to attempt different purging methods for various subgroups of ALL. Immunomodulating agents may provide additional approaches to ALL therapy. For adults with Philadelphia chromosome positive ALL with major breakpoint cluster region rearrangement, treatment with recombinant IFN-alpha has been proposed for patients who achieve a complete remission. The reduced number and decreased cytolytic activity of peripheral NK cells in patients with ALL along with the ability of lymphokine activated killer cells to lyse human leukemic blasts, has resulted in promising in vitro attempts to enhance the cell mediated cytotoxicity against leukemic blasts with interleukin-2.[32] The potential of immunomodulation is demonstrated by allogeneic bone marrow transplantation, where a graft-versus-leukemia effect has resulted in a decreased relapse rate in acute leukemia.

To assess the potential of photoradiation therapy for in vitro purging we have studied normal bone marrow and tumor cell clonogenicity in response to different light-activated compounds (fluorescent dyes). A 4-log depletion of lymphoid neoplastic cells has been achieved, but with a significantly lesser effect on myeloid, erythroid, and mixed colony-forming progenitor cells. These results demonstrate the usefulness of photoradiation for the ex-vivo treatment of lymphomatous marrow autografts.[38] Further improvements are needed in induction and consolidation therapy. Therapeutic benefit of various drugs used in treating ALL and role of mitoxantrone, Ara-c in treatment strategies needs to be developed. Better confirmation of the benefit of dose intensification, especially when used with growth factors and/or hematopoietic rescue is also needed.

CHRONIC MYELOGENOUS LEUKEMIA

PATHOPHYSIOLOGY

Chronic myelogenous leukemia (CML) is characterized cytogenetically by the presence of the Philadelphia (Ph) chromosome which usually originates from the reciprocal translocation t(9;22)(q34;q11). In the formation of the Ph chromosome, a large part of the ABL proto-oncogene is translocated from chromosome 9 onto the BCR gene in chromosome 22. This gives rise to a novel chimeric BCR-ABL gene, which encodes a 210-Kd (p210) fusion protein with prominent tyrosine kinase activity and transforming ability.[39,40] The product of the normal BCR gene is a 160-Kd (p160 BCR) cytosolic phosphoprotein, whose physiological role is not well defined. Sequences encoded by the first exon of BCR are responsible for the p160 BCR serine/threonine kinase activity. These sequences overlap the src-homology 2 (SH2)-binding regions of the BCR gene that are essential for the activation of the ABL tyrosine kinase and the transforming potential of the chimeric BCR-ABL oncogene. The central segment of BCR may be involved in the control of cell division after DNA replication. Furthermore, the C-terminus of BCR has recently been shown to have a GTPase-activating protein (GAP) activity for $p21^{rac}$, a member of the RAS family of small GTP-binding proteins which may also contribute to the pathogenesis of CML.[39-41] The mechanisms involve abnormal adhesion of the CML cell to the endothelium and alters the programmed cell death (apoptosis) of the CML granulocytes. Mice injected with BCR-ABL gene develop hematological malignancies similar to the ones observed in patients with CML.[40]

TREATMENT

High-dose chemotherapy can cause transient disappearance of Ph chromosome. Conventional drugs like hydroxyurea and busulfan decrease the number of CML cells but do not change the percent of cells which are positive for Ph chromosome.[42-44] Interferon-α treatment is able to decrease the Ph chromosome positivity but complete eradication of Ph chromosome (especially bcr-abl) is extremely rare.[44-47] Allogeneic bone marrow transplantation (BMT) is the treatment of choice for many patients with HLA-MLC compatible siblings.[48-50] The use of this treatment modality is based on the assumption that the high-dose chemoradiotherapy used as pretransplant conditioning therapy will not only eradicate the malignant clone, but will also result in a degree of host immunosuppression sufficient to prevent immunologically mediated graft rejection by the host. In vitro T-cell depletion of the donor marrow has been used successfully to prevent GVHD after allogeneic BMT, but can be associated with an increased incidence of both graft failure and leukemia relapse. Before the introduction of T-cell depletion, it was generally considered that the conditioning regimens used in patients with leukemia such as cyclophosphamide (Cy) and total body irradiation (TBI) were "ablative" with full donor chimerism being regularly observed and approximately half the patients remained in remission. More recently, it has been shown that mixed chimerism is more common after T-cell-depleted BMT and that it may predispose to graft rejection and leukemia relapse.[50,51]

National Marrow Donor Program (NMDP) has recently reviewed the data of 196 consecutive patients with CML who received unrelated donor marrow transplantation at 21 NMDP affiliated centers.[52] The median interval from the initiation of a search for an unrelated donor to bone marrow transplantation was 8.4 months (range, 1.7 to 34.6 months). Median age of the recipients was 33.3 years (4.5 to 54.5 years). Seventy-five recipients were female and 121 were male. At time of transplant, 115 patients were in chronic phase, 51 in accelerated phase, 14 in blast crisis, and 16 in a second or subsequent chronic phase. In 133 cases, donors and recipients were identical at the HLA A, B, and DR loci using standard serologic typing, and in 63 cases, there was nonidentity at one HLA locus. These patients were prepared for transplantation with a combination of high-dose chemotherapy and total body irradiation (n = 169) or with high-dose chemotherapy only (n = 27). Thirty-five patients received marrow depleted ex-vivo of T-lymphocytes, whereas 161 patients received non-T-depleted marrow. One hundred seventy-four of 196 patients engrafted (absolute neutrophil count $\geq 500/mm^3$ for three consecutive days). The median time to engraftment was 22 days (6 to 69 days). Twenty-two patients failed to engraft, and an additional 10 patients experienced late graft failure. The incidence of grades III or IV acute graft-versus-host disease (GVHD) was 0.54 ± 0.10, and that of extensive chronic GVHD was 0.52 ± 0.12. A lower incidence of both grades III and IV acute GVHD (P = .0003) and of extensive chronic GVHD (P = .01) were independently associated with use of T-depleted marrow (Figure 2). The actuarial incidence of hematologic relapse at 2 years is 0.11 ± 0.06. The two-year actuarial incidence of disease-free survival for patients transplanted in first chronic phase within one year of diagnosis is 0.45 ± 0.21, in chronic phase more than one year from diagnosis is 0.36 ± 0.11, in accelerated phase is 0.27 ± 0.12, in second or subsequent chronic phase is 0.22 ± 0.21, and in blast crisis is 0 (Figure 3). Fifteen of 55 patients transplanted at 40 to 50 years of age survive. Proportional hazards analysis revealed that transplantation with HLA-matched donor marrow (P=.01), transplantation at younger age (P=.02), and transplantation in first chronic phase (P=.04) had independent, beneficial effects on disease-free survival. Thirty-eight (50%) patients surviving at 1 year had normal activity levels (Karnofsky = 100%), whereas 31 recipients (41%) had mild impairment of activity (Karnofsky = 90% to 80%) and 7 recipients (9%) had severe impairment of activity (Karnofsky = 70% to 30%).

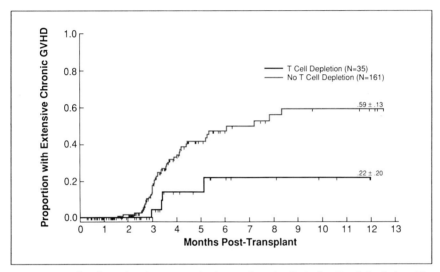

Figure 2. Results of unrelated HLA matched transplants in CML after T-cell depletion. The incidence of acute GVHD (grade III or IV) at 100 days observed in recipients of T-cell depleted bone marrow (0.2 ± 0.2) was significantly less than that observed in recipients of bone marrow not depleted of T-lymphocytes (0.6 ± 0.11) p=0.0003. The incidence of chronic GVHD is shown in this graph. At one year, recipients of T-lymphocyte-depleted bone marrow (0.22 ± 0.20) had significantly less GVHD than recipients of bone marrow not depleted of T-lymphocytes (0.59 ± 0.13)(p0.10). Reproduced with permission from Blood.[52]

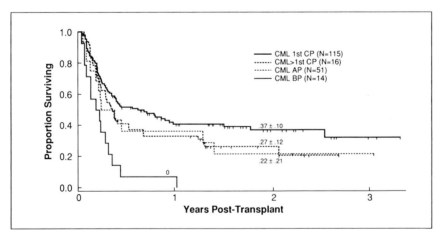

Figure 3. Results of unrelated HLA matched transplants in CML. The 2-year DFS figures and their 95% confidence intervals for patients transplanted in various stages of disease. Reproduced with permission from Blood.[52]

Development of the NMDP has facilitated the use of HLA-matched unrelated donors for marrow transplantation. This treatment modality can result in prolonged disease-free survival in some patients with CML, especially younger patients transplanted early in their disease course using donors matched at the HLA A, B, and DR loci. Further investigations are needed to decrease the high incidence of graft failure, acute and chronic GVHD.[52]

In the study of Roux et al, five patients with CML who received T-cell-depleted BM and relapsed within four years were analyzed to understand the relationship of mixed chimerism (MC) and relapse.[51] The investigators purified different populations of leukocytes and analyzed their donor/recipient origin by a method based on polymerase chain reaction amplification of mini-satellite DNA regions. The results show that before relapse, all hematopoietic recipient cells are T-cells, whereas monocytes, B, and natural killer (NK) cells are of donor origin. This observation does not appear to be specific for CML as similar results were also found in two control patients with acute myeloid leukemia (AML). At the time of (CML) relapse, recipient granulocytes, monocytes, and erythrocytes appeared and progressively replaced the respective lineages of donor origin. No other lineages seemed to be involved as B cells and NK cells remained of donor origin and no significant changes in the number of recipient T-cells were detected. In this respect, relapse of CML after ALBMT seems not to be very different from the primary disease in chronic phase before transplantation. Furthermore, it is possible that after ALBMT, an association between mixed chimerism before relapse and the (CML) relapse does exist because both phenomena are consequences of T-cell depletion of the BM graft. However, this correlation might well be indirect as the MC caused by the recipient T-cells appears to be independent of the one caused by the recurrent disease. In recent years, patients who progress after ALBMT have been treated with lymphocyte infusion.[53] Interferon-α is also being evaluated in patients with reappearance of Ph chromosome after transplantation.[54]

Recent studies have attempted to suppress Ph positive cells by combining high dose chemotherapy; enriched Ph negative cells were then harvested.[55,56] The approach is briefly detailed below: 28 patients with Ph-positive blastic phase (BP) CML or in chronic phase (CP)-CML (3 patients) and relapsed adult acute lymphoblastic leukemia (ALL) (9 patients) with cytogenetic translocation [t(8;14):2 patients; t(4;8):2 patients; t(4;11):3 patients; t(9;22):2 patients], received intensive conventional chemotherapy with idarubicin 6-8 mg/m^2 IV per day for five days with Ara-C 600-800 mg/m^2 IV over 2 hours for five days and VP-16 150 mg/m^2 IV over two hours for 3 days. During early recovery from marrow aplasia, when WBC reached 0.3-1.5x10^9/L, peripheral blood stem cells (PBSC) were collected by 4-8 leukapheresis consecutively. PBSC collected from the 2 of 3 patients with CP-CML were cytogenetically Ph-negative and were also PCR negative for BCR-ABL translocation. In 8 out of 26 BP-CML patients, PBSC were Ph-negative and in two cases PCR negative. Of the nine ALL patients, six patients lost the cytogenetic translocations, one patient died during aplasia, two patients did not have cytogenetic transformation and died in a few weeks of leukemia, and one patient out of six relapsed before transplant. After complete recovery, 15 patients (BP-CML:8 patients; CP-CML:2 patients; ALL:5 patients) were subsequently given high-dose therapy (VP-16 ± Cy+TBI in single dose) followed by reinfusion of PBSC. Both the patients in CP-CML and 5/5 patients with ALL maintain clinical and cytogenetic remission; all the patients transplanted in BP-CML relapsed 5-18 months post-transplant. It is concluded that intensive conventional chemotherapy employed in CML and ALL can lead to a precocious overshoot of cytogenetically normal PBSC.[55]

NON-HODGKIN'S LYMPHOMA

The role of molecular changes in causation and progression of lymphoma are now better understood. The role of antigen presenting cells, the mechanisms involved in presenting antigens via MLC I and MLC II molecules, how memory T-cells decide to signal the B-cells to start production of an antibody and how the B-lymphocytes switch from synthesizing one antibody to another is much better defined. Lymphoid cells have the unusual characteristic that requires rearrangement of multiple gene segments to create a functional gene. For example, the final gene products like Ig K, Ig heavy chain, T-cell receptors TcRα, TcRγ, TcRδ, etc., are arranged in discontinuous segments (a combination of variable, diverse, and constant regions) in the germline DNA. During differentiation, B- and T-cells follow systematic recombinations in order to give functional receptors and products. The variability of which segments get selected and how they rearrange accounts for the antibody diversity and spectrum of T-cell lymphocyte function.

In B-lymphocytes, heavy chain rearrangement precedes light chain gene rearrangement, and normally each cell contains one IgH and light chain. Similar changes occur in the T-cell receptor. In a normal polyclonal lymphoid cell compartment, it is very difficult to identify individual rearrangements. The switch from IgM to IgG etc. is mediated through T-cell's signals via CD-40 receptors on B-cells and requires other factors (IL-2, IL-4, IL-10, etc.). Clonal proliferation is common in lymphoproliferative disorders and offers opportunities to characterize the gene and/or the gene products related to the clonal rearrangement by DNA and RNA analysis.[5-7] Polymerase chain reaction (PCR) using specific probes (for example: bcl-2) is able to detect abnormal clones and is now widely used for diagnosis and evaluation of minimal disease.[57,58] The presence of bcl-2 delays apoptosis of normal lymphocytes and lymphomas.[6] Bone marrow involvement is very frequent in patients with lymphoma. Using clonal immunoglobulin gene rearrangements, Hu et al found evidence of lymphomatous involvement in the peripheral blood of 76% of their NHL patients, all of whom had histologically normal bone marrow biopsies.[59]

Combination chemotherapy has significantly improved the survival of patients with lymphoma. Recently, effective drugs have been combined to treat patients for a shorter duration, and the results appear very encouraging. Complete remission (CR) rates of 60% to 80% with projected five-year survival rates of 35% to 45% can be expected with effective conventional protocols (Table 1).[60] Longer follow-ups and standardized analyses of the patient's prognostic factors are necessary before the results of these trials can be fully compared. The Vancouver experience with MACOP-B, VACOP-B and the recent attempt of intermediate dose chemotherapy with hematopoietic growth factor support are reasonable avenues to explore.[61] Such analyses should also evaluate the difference in response due to the presence of various chromosomal abnormalities and the possible role of viral oncogenes in some lymphomas. Investigators have evaluated various prognostic factors, and it

Table 1. Comparison of various protocols to treat advanced disease lymphoma[60]*

Treatment	%DFS at 4 Years	% Mortality	Cost
CHOP	36.4	1	1.00
m-BACOD	34.4	5	2.26
PRO-MACE CYTOBOM	45.1	4	1.44
MACOP-B	38.8	6	1.13

*Modified from reference #60.

appears that tumor bulk, high serum lactate dehydrogenase (LDH) at presentation (may be a reflection of high tumor burden), mediastinal or abdominal mass, performance status, stage, histologic classification, bone marrow involvement, or lack of rapid response to therapy may define a group of patients with poor prognosis.[62,63] Such patients with poor prognosis lymphoma do better with upfront AUBMT in complete or partial remission.[62] Further studies with larger group of patients are needed to decide the optimum initial therapy of the patients. Especially the therapy for low grade lymphomas may have to be different from the management strategies for high grade lymphoma.

Patients with NHL who relapse after achieving a CR or are resistant to front-line chemotherapy have a poor prognosis with a minimal chance of cure with current salvage regimens. Furthermore, patients who are responsive to salvage therapy before transplant do better than patients who are transplanted when they have disease resistant to cytotoxic drugs.[62,64] Using the experience from various trials, we at MSKCC attempted to induce a CR in patients with relapsed/resistant NHL before AUBMT in an effort to decrease to toxic complications, and added VP-16 to the conditioning regimen of total body irradiation (TBI) and cyclophosphamide (CTX) to decrease the relapse rate. The results using TBI, VP-16, CTX (7% relapse rate) were better than the results when TBI, CTX (55% relapse rate) was used.[62] This observation emphasizes the importance of dose intensity of the conditioning regimen (Figure 4). The comparison of distinct AUBMT protocols between various institutions for relapsed/resistant NHL is difficult because of the marked differences in patient populations, salvage regimens, and transplant conditioning regimens.

The major determinant of survival in the MSKCC series was the remission status of the patients at the time of transplant. Patients transplanted in CR had a DFS rate of 80% while patients in PR or progressive disease (PD) had a DFS of only 60% and 11%, respectively. This observation has been reported by several investigators and reemphasized the dilemma faced in treating patients with PD: the need for more dose-intensive therapy before transplant balanced by the fact that because of intolerable toxicities, these patients are the least able to benefit from aggressive therapy. Relapse was not a major problem in this study because only three patients relapsed and no late relapses (>1 year) have occurred. The use of boost radiotherapy, TBI, VP-16, and CTX had a high early mortality (36%), especially in patients with PR and PD. These patients had a higher incidence of developing pulmonary decompensation with hemorrhage. The lysis of diseased and surrounding tissue with aggressive cytotoxic therapy and slow recovery of the normal tissue were thought to be the contributing factors for the hemorrhagic complications. Concomitant thrombocytopenia and probable or documented infections also contributed to this decompensation.[62,65,66] Several therapeutic changes can be considered to decrease toxicity: (1) early pulmonary workup including bronchoscopy and biopsy; (2) use of high-dose corticosteroids early after infectious causes of ARDS are ruled out; (3) increasing the rest period between boost radiotherapy and TBI or alter the dose or fractionation schedule of TBI; and (4) use of growth factor or chemoprotectants. Other series also report significant toxicity when such aggressive dosage of cytotoxic therapy is used. [66]

Patients transplanted in PR and PD are a poor prognostic group because they are minimally responsive or unresponsive to conventional-dose cytotoxic therapy.[67] Future strategies should concentrate on (1) further improvements in reinduction regimens to induce more patients in CR before AUBMT; (2) decreasing the toxicity without compromising the dose intensity of the conditioning regimens; and (3) use of prognostic indicators to identify this subgroup and allow the use of early AUBMT or new therapeutic strategies in this group of patients. Nine extensively pretreated low-grade lymphoma patients received TBI, VP-16 and CTX: seven are alive without disease.[62] Other series have reported improved survival in patients with low-grade lymphoma when compared with patients with intermediate- or high-grade lymphoma. This may be because of the fact that the patients with low-grade

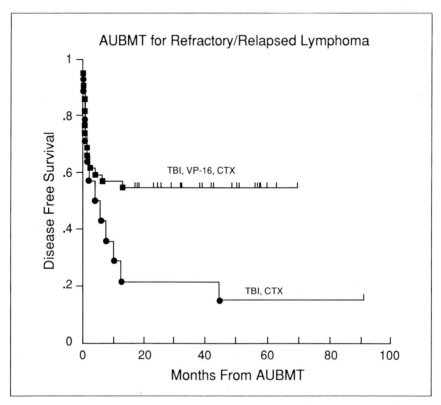

Figure 4. Comparison of the two different conditioning regimens for patients with refractory/ relapsed lymphoma. In the earlier study, patients received total body irradiation, total dose (TD) 1320 rads and CTX (TD) 120 mg/kg. Subsequently, VP-16 (TD) 750 mg/m² was added to the conditioning regimen.

lymphoma received less dose-intensive chemotherapy before AUBMT, and therefore were less likely to have toxic complications. The role of AUBMT in low-grade NHL will require more patients and a longer follow-up, especially in view of the potential of this subgroup for late relapses.

The therapeutic benefit of bone marrow purging in clinical trials for patients with lymphoma is hard to demonstrate because of various types of lymphoma, the difficulty in detecting minimal numbers of neoplastic cells in the bone marrow (exception: patients with PCR [bcl-2] positive disease[68]), and the large number of patients required for such studies. Among the various purging agents evaluated at MSKCC, we found that optimal purging was obtained with 4-HC in combination with VP-16. Therefore, we used 4-HC and VP-16 to purge the marrow of patients with a previous history of marrow involvement by lymphoma, but the patients had to have no lymphoma involvement at the time of harvest. This was done because of our assessment that these methods only eliminate minimal disease which is not detected by current technology.[62] Contrary to what is observed in NHL at diagnosis, in which marrow involvement is a poor prognostic sign associated with a high relapse rate, there is controversy concerning the prognostic significance of previous marrow involvement in AUBMT trials. The patients who received 4-HC and VP-16-purged marrow had a similar survival as those patients who received untreated marrow. Perhaps 4-HC and VP-16 purging has influenced the outcome of patients with previous history of marrow involvement (Figure 5). A longer

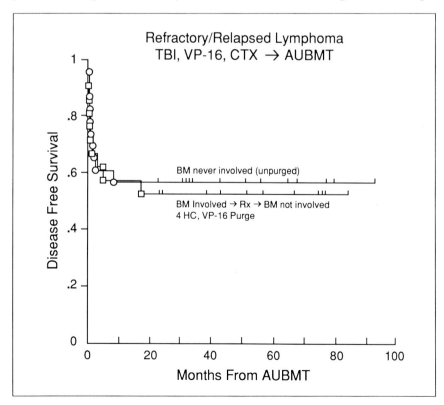

Figure 5. Comparison of patients receiving 4-HC and VP-16 purged AUBMT (for patients with previous history of BM involvement but no involvement at time of BM harvest) with patients who received unpurged AUBMT (for patients with no history of BM involvement). The conditioning regimen (TBI, VP-16, CTX) was the same for both subgroups.

follow-up and randomized clinical trials will be required to determine the significance of this observation.[62]

HODGKIN'S DISEASE

Most patients with Hodgkin's disease (HD) can be first managed with standard therapy.[64, 69] Intensive therapy with hematopoietic stem cell rescue can be considered for patients with Hodgkin's disease only if they are refractory or fail first attempt with conventional combination chemotherapy within one year or have second or subsequent relapse. Autologous SCT is preferred over allogeneic especially if the BM is not involved. Often publications combine the results of BMT for HD with those of patients being treated for lymphoma.[69,70] No reliable scientifically proven purging method is available and we need to understand more about the biology of Hodgkin's disease.

MULTIPLE MYELOMA

Usually patients with multiple myeloma (MM) are older and optimum conditioning regimen for in vivo treatment is not yet established.[71,72] Melphalan has been used most often. Various methods for purging BM have been developed with promising results.[73-76]

REFERENCES

1. McCulloch EA: Stem cells in normal and leukemic hemopoiesis (Henry Stratton Lecture). Blood 1983; 62:1-13.
2. Dexter TM, Allen TD, Lajtha LG: Conditions controlling the proliferation of haemopoietic stem cells in vitro. J Cell Physiol 1976; 91:335-344.
3. Nowell PC: Chromosomal approaches to hematopoietic oncogenesis. Stem Cells 1993; 11:9-19.
4. Nichols J, Nimer SD: Transcription factors, translocations, and leukemia. Blood 1992; 80:2953-2963.
5. Leder P, Battey J, Lenoir G, Moulding C, Murphy W, Potter H, Stewart T, Taub R: Translocations among antibody genes in human cancer. Science 1983; 222:765-771.
6. Campana D, Coustan-Smith, Manabe A, Buschle M, Raimondi SC, Behm, FG, Ashmum R, Arico M, Biondi A, Pui C-H: Prolonged survival of B-lineage acute lymphoblastic leukemia cells is accompanied by overexpression of bcl-2 protein. Blood 1993; 81:1025-1031.
7. Rowley JD: Molecular cytogenetics: Rosetta stone for understanding cancer —Twenty-ninth G.H.A. Clowes Memorial Award Lecture. Cancer Res 1990; 50:3816-3825.
8. Liesveld JL, Winslow JM, Frediani KE, Ryan DH, Abboud CN: Expression of integrins and examination of their adhesive function in normal and leukemic hematopoietic cells. Blood 1993; 81:112-121.
9. Srour EF, Brandt JE, Briddell RA, Grigsby S, Leemhuis T, Hoffman R: Long-term generation and expansion of human primitive hematopoietic progenitor cells in vitro. Blood 1993; 81:661-669.
10. Lowenberg B, Touw IP: Hematopoietic growth factors and their receptors in acute leukemia. Blood 1993; 81:281-292.
11. Tighe JE, Daga A, Calabi F: Translocation breakpoints are clustered on

both chromosome 8 and chromosome 21 in the t(8;21) of acute myeloid leukemia. Blood 1993; 81:592-596.

12. Degos L: Approaches for an explanation of the differentiating effect of all trans retinoic acid in acute promyelocytic leukemia. Leukemia 1992; 6(Suppl 4):44-46.

13. Mayer RJ: Current chemotherapeutic treatment approaches to the management of previously untreated adults with de novo acute myelogenous leukemia. Semin Oncol 1987; 14:384-396.

14. Berman E, Heller G, Santorsa J, McKenzie S, Gee TS, Kempin S, Gulati SC, Andreeff M, Kolitz J, Gabrilove J, Reich L, Mayer K, Keefe D, Trainor K, Schluger A, Penenber D, Raymond V, O'Reilly R, Jhanwar S, Young C, Clarkson B: Results of a randomized trial comparing idarubicin and cytosine arabinoside with daunorubicin and cytosine arabinoside in adult patients with newly diagnosed acute myelogenous leukemia. Blood 1991; 77:1666-1674.

15. Preisler H, Davis RB, Kirshner J, Dupre E, Richards F III, Hoagland HC, Kopel S, Levy RN, Carey R, Schulman P, Gottlieb AJ, McIntyre OR: Comparison of three remission induction regimens and two postinduction strategies for the treatment of acute nonlymphocytic leukemia: A cancer and Leukemia Group B Study. Blood 1987; 69:1141-1449.

16. Young JW, Papadopoulos EB, Cunningham I, Castro-Malaspina H, Flomenberg N, Carabasi MH, Gulati SC, Brochstein JA, Heller G, Black P, Collins NH, Shank B, Kernan NA, O'Reilly RJ: T-cell-depleted allogeneic bone marrow transplantation in adults with acute nonlymphocytic leukemia in first remission. Blood 1992; 79:3380-3387.

17. McGlave PB, Haake RJ, Bostrom BC, Brunning R, Hurd DD, Kim TH, Nesbit ME, Vercellotti GM, Weisdorf D, Woods WG, Ramsay NKC, Kersey JH: Allogeneic bone marrow transplantation for acute nonlymphocytic leukemia in first remission. Blood 1988; 72:1512-1517.

18. Cassileth PA, Andersen J, Lazarus HM, Colvin OM, Bennett JM, Stadtmauer EA, Kaizer H, Weiner RS, Edelstein M, Oken MM: Autologous bone marrow transplant in acute myeloid leukemia in first remission. J Clin Oncol 1993; 11:314-319.

19. Labopin M, Gorin NC: Autologous bone marrow transplantation in 2502 patients with acute leukemia in Europe: a retrospective study. Leukemia 1992; 6(Suppl 4):95-99.

20. Gulati SC, Acaba L, Yahalom J, Reich L, Motzer R, Crown J, Doherty M, Clarkson B, Berman E, Atzpodien J, Andreef M, Gee TS: Autologous bone marrow transplantation for acute myelogenous leukemia using 4-hydroperoxycyclophosphamide and VP-16 purged bone marrow. Bone Marrow Transplantation 1992; 10:129-134.

21. Henon P: New developments in peripheral blood stem cell transplants. Leukemia 1992; 6(Suppl 4):106-109.

22. Gulati SC, Lemoli RM, Acaba L, Igarashi T, Wasserheit C, Fraig M: Purging in autologous and allogeneic bone marrow transplantation. Current Opinion in Onc 1992; 4:264-271.

23. Lemoli RM, Gasparetto C, Scheinberg DA, Moore MAS, Clarkson BD, Gulati SC: Autologous bone marrow transplantation in acute myelog-

enous leukemia: In vitro treatment with myeloid-specific monoclonal antibodies and drugs in combination. Blood 1991; 77:1829-1836.

24. Ranson MR, Scarffe JH, Morgenstern GR, Chang J, Anderson H, Deakin DP, Oppenheim B, Heron D, Ryder D: Post consolidation therapy for adult patients with acute myeloid leukemia. British Journal of Haematology 1991; 79:162-169.

25. Ramsay NKC, Kersey JH. Indications for marrow transplantation in acute lymphoblastic leukemia. Blood 1990, 75:815-818.

26. Kantarijan HM, Estey EH, O'Brien S, Anaissie E, Beran M, Rios MB, Keating MJ, Gutterman J: Intensive chemotherapy with mitoxantrone and high-dose cytosine arabinoside followed by granulocyte-macrophage colony-stimulating factor in the treatment of patients with acute lympho-cytic leukemia. Blood 1992, 79:876-881.

27. Gulati SC, Gaynor J, Esseesse I, Gee TS, Little C, Andreeff M, Berman E, Kempin S, Clarkson B: Use of prognostic factors in deciding therapy for adult acute lymphoblastic leukemia: new approaches at Memorial Sloan-Kettering Cancer Center. Bone Marrow Transplantation 1989; 4 (Suppl 1):86-89.

28. Walters R, Kantarjian HM, Keating MJ, Estey EH, Trujillo J, Cork A, McCredie KB, Freireich EJ: The importance of cytogenetic studies in adult acute lymphocytic leukemia. American J of Med 1990, 89:579-584.

29. Pozzatti R, Vogel J, Jay G. The human T-lymphotropic virus type I tax gene can cooperate with the ras oncogene to induce neoplastic transfor-mation of cells. Molecul and Cellul Biol 1990, 10:413-417.

30. Secker-Walker LM, Craig JM, Hawkins JM, Hoffbrand AV. Philadel-phia positive acute lymphoblastic leukemia in adults: age distribution, bcr breakpoint and prognostic significance. Leukemia 1991, 5:196-199.

31. Fenaux P, Jonveaux P, Quiquandon I, Preudhomme C, Lai JL, Vanrumbeke M, Loucheux-Lefebvre MH, Bauters F, Berger R, Kerckaert JP: Mutations of the p53 gene in B-cell lymphoblastic acute leukemia: a report on 60 cases. Leukemia 1992, 6:42-46.

32. Foa R, Guarini A, Tos AG, Cardona S, Fierro MT, Meloni G, Tosti S, Mandelli F, Gavosto F: Peripheral blood and bone marrow immunophenotypic and functional modifications induced in acute leukemia patients treated with interleukin 2: evidence of in vivo lympho-kine activated killer cell generation. Cancer Res 1991, 51:964-968.

33. Carey PJ, Proctor SJ, Taylor P, Hamilton PJ: Autologous bone marrow transplantation for high-grade lymphoid malignancy using melphalan/irradiation conditioning without marrow purging or cryopreservation. Blood 1991; 77:1593-1598.

34. Uckun FM, Kersey JH, Vallera DA, Ledbetter JA, Weisdorf D, Myers DE, Haake R, Ramsay NKC: Autologous bone marrow transplantation in high-risk remission T-lineage acute lymphoblastic leukemia using immunotoxins plus 4-HC for marrow purging. Blood 1990; 76:1723-1733.

35. Ochs J, Brecher ML, Mahoney D, Vega R, Pollock GH, Buchanan GR, Whitehead VM, Ravindranath Y, Freeman AI: Recombinant interferon alfa given before and in combination with standard chemotherapy in

children with acute lymphoblastic leukemia in first marrow relapse: a Pediatric Oncology Group pilot study. J Clin Oncol 1991, 9:777-782.

36. Kersey J, Weisdorf D, Nesbit M, LeBien T, Woods W, McGlave P, Kim T, Vallera D, Goldman A, Bostrom B, Hurd D, Ramsay N: Comparison of autologous and allogeneic bone marrow transplantation for treatment of high-risk refractory acute lymphoblastic leukemia. New England Journal of Medicine 1987; 317:461-467.

37. Ramsay N, Kersey J, Nesbit M, McGlave P, Haake R, McCullough J, Weisdorf D: Unrelated donor bone marrow transplantation for patients with high risk acute lymphoblastic leukemia. Blood 1992; 80 (Suppl 1):246.

38. Gulati SC, Acaba L, Maslak P, Phillips J, Duensing S: Acute lymphoblastic leukemia: present and future. Leukemia 1992; 6(Suppl 4):52-55.

39. Maru Y, Witte ON: The BCR gene encodes a novel serine/threonine kinase activity within a single exon. Cell 1991; 67:459-468.

40. Daley GQ, van Etten RA, Baltimore D: Induction of chronic myelogenous leukemia in mice by the P210 bcr/abl gene of the Philadelphia chromosome. Science 1990; 247:824-830.

41. Melo JV, Gordon DE, Cross NCP, Goldman JM: The abl-bcr fusion gene is expressed in chronic myeloid leukemia. Blood 1993; 81:158-165.

42. Hehlmann R, Heimpel H, Griesshammer M, Kolb HJ, Heinze B, Hossfeld DK, Wickramanayake PD, Essers U, Thiele J, Georgii A, Ansari H, Hochhaus A, Hasford J: Chronic myelogenous leukemia: Recent developments in prognostic evaluation and chemotherapy. Leukemia 1992; 6(Suppl 3):110-114.

43. Wandl UB, Kloke O, Nagel-Hiemke M, Moritz T, Becher R, Opalka B, Holtkamp W, Bartels H, Seeber S, Niederle N: Combination therapy with interferon α-2b plus low-dose interferon gamma in pretreated patients with Ph+ chronic myelogenous leukemia. British J of Haematol 1992; 81:516-519.

44. Tura S, Russo D, Zaffa E, Fiacchini M, Baccarani M: A prospective comparison of α-IFN and conventional chemotherapy in Ph+ chronic myeloid leukemia. Clinical and cytogenetic results at 2 years in 322 patients. Haematol 1992; 77:204-214.

45. Talpaz M, Kantarjian H, Kurzrock R, Trujillo JM, Gutterman JU: Interferon α produces sustained cytogenetic responses in chronic myelogenous leukemia Philadelphia chromosome + patients. Ann Intern Med 1991; 114:532-538.

46. Dhingra K, Talpaz M, Kantarjian H, Ku S, Rothberg J, Gutterman JU, Kurzrock R: Appearance of acute leukemia-associated P190 BCR/ABL in chronic myelogenous leukemia may correlate with disease progression. Leukemia 1991; 5:191-195.

47. Lee M-S, Kantarjian H, Talpaz M, Freireich EJ, Deisseroth A, Trujillo JM, Stass SA: Detection of minimal residual disease by polymerase chain reaction in philadelphia chromosome-positive chronic myelogenous leukemia following interferon therapy. Blood 1992; 79:1920-1923.

48. Thomas ED, Clift RA, Fefer A, Appelbaum FR, Beatty P, Bensinger WI, Buckner CD, Cheever MA, Deeg HJ, Doney K, Flournoy N, Greenberg P, Hansen JA, martin P, McGuttin R, Ramberg R, Sanders JE, Singer

JW, Stewart P, Storb R, Sullivan K, Weiden PL, Witherspoon R: Marrow transplantation for the treatment of chronic myelogenous leukemia. Ann Intern Med 1986; 104:155-163.

49. Cunningham I, Castro-Malaspina H, Flomenberg N, Gulati SC, Shank B, Collins N, Keever C, O'Reilly RJ: Improved results of bone marrow transplantation for chronic myelogenous leukemia using marrow depleted of T-cells by soybean lectin agglutination and E-rosette depletion. Progress in Bone Marrow Transplantation Alan R. Liss, Inc. 1987; 359-363.

50. Mackinnon S, Hows JM, Goldman JM: Induction of in vitro graft-versus-leukemia activity following bone marrow transplantation for chronic myeloid leukemia. Blood 1990; 76:2037-2045.

51. Roux E, Abdi K, Speiser D, Helg C, Chapuis B, Jeannet M, Roosnek E: Characterization of mixed chimerism in patients with chronic myeloid leukemia transplanted with T-cell-depleted bone marrow: Involvement of different hematologic lineages before and after relapse. Blood 1993; 81:243-248.

52. McGlave P, Bartsch G, Anasetti C, Ash R, Beatty P, Gajewski J, Kernan NA: Unrelated donor marrow transplantation therapy for chronic myelogenous leukemia: Initial experience of the National Marrow Donor Program. Blood 1993; 81:543-550.

53. Bar BMAM, Schattenberg A, Mensink EJBM, Guerts Van Kessel A, Smetsers TFCM, Knops GHJN, Linders EHP, De Witte T: Donor leukocyte infusions for chronic myeloid leukemia relapsed after allogeneic bone marrow transplantations. J Clin Oncology 1993; 11:513-519.

54. Higano CS, Raskind WH, Singer JW: Use of α interferon for the treatment of relapse of chronic myelogenous leukemia in chronic phase after allogeneic bone marrow transplantation. Blood 1992; 80:1437-1442.

55. Carella AM, Policardo N, Raffo MR, Podesta M, Carlier P, Valbonesi M, Lercari G, Vitale V, Gallamini A: Intensive conventional chemotherapy can lead to a precocious overshoot of cytogenetically normal blood stem cells (BSC) in chronic myeloid leukemia and acute lymphoblastic leukemia. Leukemia 1992; 6(Suppl 4):120-123.

56. Leemhuis T, Leibowitz D, Cox G, Silver R, Srour EF, Tricot G, Hoffman R: Identification of BCR/ABL-negative primitive hematopoietic progenitor cells within chronic myeloid leukemia marrow. Blood 1993; 81:801-807.

57. Chleq-Deschamps CM, LeBrun DP, Huie P, Besnier DP, Warnke RA, Sibley RK, Cleary ML: Topographical dissociation of BCL-2 messenger RNA and protein expression in human lymphoid tissues. Blood 1993; 81:293-298.

58. Vaux DL, Weissman IL, Kim SK: Prevention of programmed cell death in caenorhabditis elegans by human bcl-2. Science 1992; 258:1955-1957.

59. Hu E, Thompson J, Horning S, Trela M, Lowder J, Levy R, Sklar J: Detection of B-cell lymphoma in peripheral blood by DNA hybridization. Lancet 1985; 2:1092-1094.

60. Fisher RI, Gaynor E, Dahlberg S, Mize EM, Oken MM: A phase III

comparison of CHOP vs m-BACOD vs ProMACE-CytaBOM vs MACOP-B in patients with intermediate or high-grade non-Hodgkin's lymphoma: Preliminary results of SWOG-8516 (Intergroup 0067), the national high priority lymphoma study. Proc Am Soc Clin Oncol 1992; 11:1067.

61. O'Brien J, O'Keefe P, Roistacher N, Offit K, Norton L, Bertino J, Filippa D, Castellino R, Straus D, Portlock C: NHL-15 protocol for diffuse aggressive lymphomas: A dose intense regimen of doxorubicin, vincristine, and cyclophosphamide. Blood 1992: 80(Suppl 1):620.

62. Gulati SC, Yahalom J, Acaba L, Reich L, Motzer R, Crown J, Toia M, Igarashi T, Lemoli R, Hanninen E, Doherty M: Treatment of patients with relapsed and resistant non-hodgkin's lymphoma using total body irradiation, etoposide, and cyclophosphamide and autologous bone marrow transplantation. J Clin Oncol 1992; 10:936-941.

63. Coeffier B, Gisselbrecht C, Vose JM, Tilley H, Herbrecht R, Bosly A, Armitage JO: Prognostic factors in aggressive malignant lymphomas: Description and validation of a prognostic index that could identify patients requiring a more intensive therapy. J Clin Oncol 1991; 9:211-219.

64. DeVita VT, Hubbard SM, Longo DL: The chemotherapy of lymphoma: Looking back, moving forward. The Richard and Hinda Rosenthal foundation award lecture. Can Res 1987; 47:5810-5824.

65. Jules-Elysee K, Stover DE, Yahalom J, White DA, Gulati SC: Pulmonary complications in lymphoma patients treated with high-dose therapy and autologous bone marrow transplantation. Am Rev Respir Dis 1992; 146:485-491.

66. Robbins RA, Linder J, Stahl MG, Thompson AB III, Haire W, Kessinger A, Armitage JO, Arneson M, Woods G, Vaughan WP, Rennard SI: Diffuse alveolar hemorrhage in autologous bone marrow transplant recipients. Am J Med 1989; 87:511-518.

67. Philip T, Chauvin J, Armitage JO, Bron D, Hagenbeek A, Biron P, Spitzer G, Velasquez W, Weisenburger DD, Fernandez-Ranada J, Somers R, Rizzoli V, Harousseau JL, Sotto JJ, Cahn JY, Guilhot F, Biggs J, Sonneveld P, Misset JL, Manna A, Jagannath S, Guglielmi C, Chevreau C, Delmer A, Santini G, Coiffier B: Parma International Protocol: Pilot study of DHAP followed by involved-field radiotherapy and BEAC with autologous bone marrow transplantation. Blood 1991; 77:1587-1592.

68. Gribben JG, Freedman AS, Neuberg D, Roy CD, Blake KW, Sunhee DW, Grossbard ML, Rabinowe SN, Coarl F, Freeman GJ, Ritz J, Nadler LM: Immunologic purging of marrow assessed by PCR before autologous bone marrow transplantation of B-cell lymphoma. NEJM 1991; 325:1525-1533.

69. DeVita VT, Hubbard SM: Hodgkin's disease. N Engl J Med 1993; 328:560-565.

70. Gulati SC, Yahalom J, Portlock C: Autologous bone marrow transplantation. Curr Probl Cancer 1991; 15:1-57.

71. Second International Workshop on Myeloma: Advances in biology and therapy of multiple myeloma. Can Research 1989; 49:7172-7175.

72. Jagannath S, Vesole DH, Glenn L, Crowley J, Barlogie B: Low-risk

intensive therapy for multiple myeloma with combined autologous bone marrow and blood stem cell support. Blood 1992; 80:1666-1672.

73. Shimazaki C, Wisniewski, Scheinberg DA, Atzpodien J, Strife A, Gulati SC, Fried J, Wisniewolski R, Wang CY, Clarkson BD: Elimination of myeloma cells from bone marrow by using monoclonal antibodies and magnetic immunobeads. Blood 1988; 72:1248-1254.

74. Shimazaki C, Gulati SC, Atzpodien J, Fried J, Colvin OM, Clarkson BD: Ex-vivo treatment of myeloma cells by 4-HC and VP-16-213. Acta Haematologica 1988; 80:17-22.

75. Shimazaki C, Inaba T, Murakami S, Fujita N, Nakagawa M, Gulati SC, Fried J, Clarkson BD, Wisniewski, Wang CY: Purging of myeloma cells from bone marrow using monoclonal antibodies and magnetic immunobeads in combination with 4-HC. Bone Marrow Purging and Processing 1990; 311-319.

76. Tazzari PL, Battelli MG, Abbondanza A, Dinota A, Rizzi, Gobbi M, Stirpe F: Targeting of a plasma cell line with a conjugate containing xanthine oxidase and the monoclonal antibody 62B1[1]. Transplantation 1989; 48:119-122.

RESULTS OF PURGING
IN SOLID TUMORS

Solid tumors which most frequently have bone marrow involvement are breast cancer, neuroblastoma, prostate cancer, Ewing's sarcoma, melanoma and small cell lung cancer. High dose chemotherapy with intent of stem cell transplantation (SCT) can be planned for diseases where a higher dose-response benefit is expected. For this reason, no significant trials suggesting clinical benefit of high dose therapy with SCT have been published for prostate cancer and melanoma (efficacy of the suitable drug needs to be established first). Various investigators have developed purging conditions for breast cancer, neuroblastoma, and Ewing's sarcoma.[1-5] Some of the results are briefly detailed in this chapter.

BREAST CANCER

Bone marrow is involved in one-fourth of the patients with primary breast cancer. The incidence increases to 40-60% in patients with Stage IV breast cancer. In one study, the number of sites of bone metastases by bone scan correlated with marrow involvement by histological stains. Patients with one, two, three or greater than three had 44, 48, 73 and 94% positivity, respectively, for involvement of the bone marrow.[6]

Preclinical experiments have shown a 4-5 log depletion of breast cancer cells (from a mixture of breast cancer cell live and normal bone marrow) by using SBA-linked magnetic microspheres with 4-HC.[7] Antibodies against breast cancer cells (LICR-LOW-Fib 75, DF-3) have been conjugated to toxins and have shown 1.6 to 2.8 log reduction of the breast cancer cell lines with a 30% decrease in CFU-GM growth of the human bone marrow treated under similar conditions. A purging method utilizing five different antibodies against breast cancer cause 3-5 log depletion of clonogenic breast cancer cells.[3,9] In similar experiments, 4-HC causes a 2.5 log reduction of malignant cells. Sequential treatment resulted in 4.5 log elimination of breast cancer cells.[10]

Phase I clinical studies utilizing 4-HC alone, antibody or a combination with immunomagnetic method and toxin conjugated LICR-LON-75 antibody showed good hematopoietic engraftment.[11] Studies to prove the clinical benefit of purged bone marrow need to be performed. Better understanding of possible oncogenes involved in breast cancer may change the future design of purging for this disease. Several groups use unpurged PBSC with the hope that the PBSC will have less risk of contamination with breast cancer. However, this hypothesis requires scientific proof. The studies are difficult because minimal residual disease is hard to diagnose in patients with breast cancer. The role of AUBMT for patients with breast cancer is part of several clinical studies. Furthermore, attempts are being made to compare the clinical benefit of AUBMT versus conventional therapy.[12]

NEUROBLASTOMA

Neuroblastoma (NB) is the most common extracranial solid tumor of childhood. Infants under one year of age and children with localized, resectable tumors have a good prognosis.[13] Unfortunately, more than 60% of the patients present with disseminated disease at the time of diagnosis. Although conventional chemotherapy produces remission in about 50% of these patients, responses are typically short-lived, and long-term disease-free survival rates of patients with advanced neuroblastoma remain less than 10%. Conventional multimodality therapy produced 10% of long-term disease-free survival in patients with poor-risk neuroblastoma. This fact, plus laboratory and clinical data indicating dose-responsiveness of neuroblastoma to alkylating agents, prompted trials of very high-dose melphalan-based treatments alone[14] or with total body irradiation (TBI)[15]. To reverse marrow aplasia, most groups infused autologous bone marrow; usually after ex vivo immunologic[16] or pharmacologic[17-20] purging of possible residual neuroblasts.

In one study, a panel of seven antineuroblastoma monoclonal antibodies were evaluated for purging.[20] They demonstrated that 3 logs of neuroblastoma cells could be consistently removed from bone marrow with the immunomagnetic purging technique. In depletion experiments with Hoechst dye-labeled neuroblastoma cells, Kemshead et al demonstrated that no residual neuroblasts could be identified in marrow samples containing 1-5% of the tumor cells before purging.[21] Clinical trials utilizing the immunomagnetic purging methods are ongoing. Initial results suggested that applying myeloablative cytoreduction regimens immediately after induction therapy prolonged survival of patients with stage IV neuroblastoma. While local boost radiation appeared beneficial, the importance of TBI to treatment efficacy is unclear. Comparable results were obtained by Philip et al[22] when melphalan was used alone or in combination with TBI.

In the first clinical trial at Memorial Sloan-Kettering Cancer Center (MSKCC),[17] 28 patients who were diagnosed with neuroblastoma at more than 12 months of age were treated with melphalan 180 mg/m^2 (n = 6) or 240 mg/m^2 (n - 22) to consolidate remissions of Stage IV disease or to control refractory disease. Twenty-four patients also received dianhydrogalactitol 180 to 240 mg/m^2, and 11 received total body irradiation 450 to 600 cGy. Autologous bone marrow transplantation (AUBMT) was performed with marrow that was unpurged (n = 2) or purged ex vivo (n = 26) with 6-hydroxydopamine (6-OHDA) 20 mcg/ml plus ascorbate 200 mcg/ml. The median time to an absolute neutrophil count of 500 mcg/ml was 21 days and to self-sustaining platelet counts more than 20,000/mcl, 28 days. One patient required infusion of unpurged reserve marrow. Two groups of patients underwent AUBMT: (1) 17 patients (Group I) who were in first remission a median of 7 months after diagnosis; and (2) 11 patients (Group II) who had refractory disease or were in second remission. For Group I, event-free survival was 29% at 12 months and 6% at 24 months post-AUBMT. All Group II patients died of disease or AUBMT-related toxicity. Overall, of the 28 patients, one is a long-term relapse-free survivor; five died of AUBMT-related toxicity; ten patients with tumors present at AUBMT had progressive disease within six months of AUBMT; and 12 patients with no measurable disease at AUBMT relapsed 4 to 32 (median 12) months post-AUBMT. Among the latter, six relapses involved the primary site, and six were restricted to distant sites. These results are in agreement with the long-term outcome in other series and suggest that for patients with neuroblastoma, high-dose melphalan cannot be relied on to ablate residual disease or to salvage patients with refractory tumors. In addition, the pattern of relapse in several patients could be explained by infusion of incompletely purged autografts; this would support recent laboratory evidence that 6-OHDA/ascorbate is a suboptimal purging method.[18,19] In the subsequent study at MSKCC,[19] myeloablative treatment intensification in 25 patients diagnosed when older than 12 months of age with Stage IV neuroblastoma included sequential delivery of cisplatin 120 mg/m^2 x 1, hyperfractionated radiation (2,100 cGy) to the primary site and adjacent lymph nodes, carmustine (BCNU 200 mg/m^2 x 1, melphalan 60 mg/m^2/d x 3 (n = 13) or thiotepa 300 mg/m^2/d x 3 (n = 12), and etoposide (VP-16) 300 mg/m^2/d x 3. Seventy-two hours after the last dose of VP-16, histologically tumor-free and 4-hydroperoxycyclophosphamide (4-HC; 100 mcmol)-purged autologous bone marrow (AUBMT) was infused. Acute toxicities included grade 3 to 4 oral mucositis, grade 1 to 2 diarrhea and fevers. No patient required infusion of unpurged reserve autografts. At AUBMT, 16 patients (Group I) were progression-free 6.5 to 14 months (median, 9 months) from diagnosis: seven remain progression-free 20 to 46 months (median, 39 months) off therapy, six relapsed 4 to 17 months post-AUBMT, and three died of toxicity (candidiasis, metabolic derangement, and venoocclusive disease [VOD]). The event-free survival of Group I patients is 44% at 24 months post-AUBMT. Nine patients (Group II) were in second remission at AUBMT, including three who had relapsed after other transplant procedures: two are progression-free 24 and 41 months off therapy, four relapsed 3 to 12 months post-AUBMT, and three died of toxicity (aspergillosis, hemorrhagic cystitis, VOD). Only 1 of 10 relapses involved the primary site, suggesting a beneficial effect of local radiation. In terms of survival or toxicity, an advantage for melphalan or thiotepa was not evident.[19] Regimens described above may prolong the survival of selected patients with poor-risk neuroblastoma, but concerns over late relapses and toxicity mandate continuing efforts to devise alternative, less risky, and more clearly beneficial approaches for definitive ablation of neuroblastoma.[17-23]

Future trials may utilize the effectiveness of IL-2 activated natural killer cells in treatment of neuroblastoma. Preclinical experiments have shown ex vivo sensitivity of continuously cultured neuroblastoma cells from three different patients towards interleukin-2-induced cell-mediated cytotoxicity. A mean (± SD) target cell lysis (4 h ^{51}Cr release) of 49 ± 11, 46 ± 8, and 32 ± 11% in SMS-SAN, LAN-N-1, and SKK-N-BE2 cell lines, respectively, was achieved when neuroblastoma cells were cocultured at an effector-to-target (E:T) ratio of 50:1 with peripheral blood mononuclear cells (PBMC) that had been preincubated for four days in the presence of recombinant interleukin-2 (rIL-2; 100 U/ml).[24] Such immunomodulation can be used to purge the BM or can be used post-transplant to help decrease the relapse rate.

EWING'S SARCOMA

Ewing's sarcoma (ES) is the second most common malignant bone tumor; it occurs mainly in adolescents and young adults. Significant advances have been made for the treatment of localized ES and long-term survival rates of 50-80% have been reported with multimodal treatments.[25,26] However, the prognosis of metastatic and relapsed ES patients remains poor. AUBMT has been used for the treatment of relapsed ES,[27,28] as well as a consolidation therapy for poor prognosis ES.[3,29] Bone marrow purging may have an important role in the ultimate success of AUBMT in ES, since significant numbers of ES patients have BM involvement.[3,29] In vitro effects of a variety of chemotherapeutic agents on two established ES cell lines (ES-5838 and ES-A4573) and marrow colony-forming unit-granulocyte macrophage (CFU-GM) were evaluated. 4-HC, at 100 mcM produced complete inhibition (>5 log) of clonogenic growth of both ES cell lines, and spared 6.9% of normal CFU-GM growth. Etoposide (VP-16), at 100 mcM produced 3-3.5 log inhibition of ES cell lines and complete inhibition of CFU-GM growth. Adriamycin (ADR) and vincristine (VCR) were more cytotoxic to ES-5838 cells than ES-A4573 cells. ADR at 1 mcM produced 99.7% inhibition of ES-5838 cells, 92.2% of ES-A4573 cells, and 86% inhibition of CFU-GM. VCR at 1 mcM produced 98.6% inhibition of ES-5838 cells, only 43.7% of ES-A4573 cells, and 75% inhibition of CFU-GM growth. The data is presented in Figure 1. Addition of verapamil did not enhance VCR cytotoxicity of ES cell lines. These studies indicate that 4-HC may be a useful agent for purging metastatic ES cells from the bone marrow for autologous marrow transplantation.[29] 4-HC is now being evaluated for purging in clinical trials.

It has recently been shown that natural killer (NK) and lyphokine (IL-2)-activated killer (LAK) cells can be generated with cytotoxicity towards cultured ES cells from three different patients. Target cell lysis was measured in a 4-hour ^{51}Cr radioisotope release assay. At an E:T ratio of 50:1, the mean ($\pm$ 1 SD) cytolysis by fresh purified large granular lymphocytes (NK cells) was 20 $\pm$ 8, 25 $\pm$ 2, and 21 $\pm$ 3% in ES cell lines 6647, 5838, and A4573, respectively. Under identical conditions, NK cells lysed 56 $\pm$ 7% of K562 (a standard NK target), and 3 $\pm$ 3% of Daudi (a standard NK-resistant LAK target). When compared to fresh unseparated peripheral blood mononuclear cells (PBMC), purified NK cells did not exhibit an enhanced cytotoxic reactivity against either ES target. In contrast, LAK cells, i.e., PBMC that were preincubated for four days in the presence of rIL-2, were highly cytotoxic against all three ES targets. LAK activity was dependent on the concentration of rIL-2 used in PBMC cultures. Optimum cell-mediated toxicity against the standard LAK target Daudi (99 $\pm$ 10% cytolysis at 50:1 E:T ratio) was achieved at rIL-2 concentrations of 1,000 U/ml. LAK cells grown under these conditions were also effective against ES cells. At an E:T ratio of 50:1, 86 $\pm$ 16, 85 $\pm$ 16, and 67 $\pm$ 13% inhibition was observed in 6647, 5838, and A4573 cells, respectively, as compared to 17 $\pm$ 10, 19 $\pm$ 15, and 29 $\pm$ 11% cytolysis by fresh uninduced PBMC. These results suggest that rIL-2-induced LAK-type immune effector cells may be of some therapeutic value in the purging and post-transplant management of poor prognosis ES.[30]

SMALL CELL LUNG CANCER

Monoclonal antibodies highly specific towards small cell lung cancer

(SCLC) have shown improvement in detection of minimal disease. It now appears that SCLC involves BM in 50-80% of the patients.[3,31] Immunomagnetic purging methods have been tested. In one study, specific antibodies SCCL-175, TES-4 (specific towards SCLC) and HNK-1 (reacts with SCLC on NK cells) and other Ab were evaluated. The reactivity of this panel of mAb with two SCCL cell lines and normal bone marrow and the ability of the mAb and immunomagnetic beads to eliminate the SCCL cells from a mixture of 90% normal bone marrow cells and 10% SCCL cells. The mAb and immunomagnetic beads removed 4 to 5 log of SCCL cells in the model system. The immunomagnetic separation was not significantly toxic to the normal hematopoietic progenitor cells, as determined by bone marrow colony-forming units.[32]

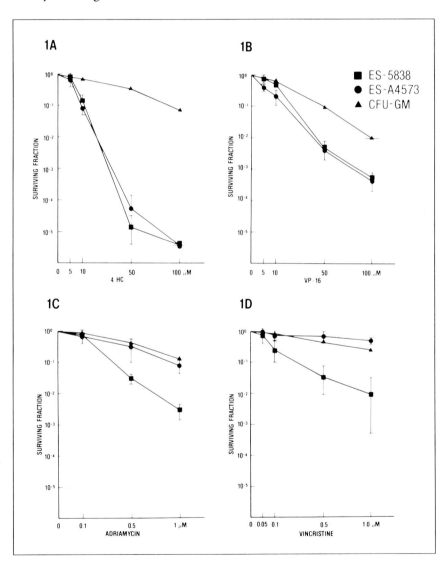

Figure 1. Effect of various cytotoxic drugs on Ewing's sarcoma cell lines and normal bone marrow colony forming units - granulocyte-macrophage. Reproduced with permission from Cancer Investigations.[29]

The results suggest that the mAb and immunomagnetic beads could safely and effectively purge SCCL cells from the bone marrow for AUBMT following high dose chemotherapy. In another study, WR-2721 (radioprotectant) and MC-540 (phototherapy) were able to eliminate SCLC selectively.[33] Some of the approaches describes above can now be considered for clinical trials.

REFERENCES

1. Gross S, Gee AP, Worthington-White DA, eds: Progress in clinical and biological research, bone marrow purging and processing. Vol 333 Alan R. Liss Publisher, 1990.

2. Gulati SC, Lemoli RM, Acaba L, Igarashi T, Wasserheit C, Mustafa F: Purging in autologous and allogeneic bone marrow transplantation. Current Opinion in Oncology 1992, 4:264-271.

3. Shpall EJ, Johnson C, Hami L: Bone marrow purging, In: Armitage JO and Antman KH, ed. High dose cancer therapy. Baltimore, Maryland: Williams and Wilkins, 1992; 249-275.

4. Morecki S, Pavlotsky S, Margel S, Slavin S: Purging breast cancer cells in preparation for autologous bone marrow transplantation. Bone Marrow Transplant 1987; 1:357-363.

5. Reynolds PC, Seeger RC, Co DD, Black AT, Wells J, Ugelstad J: Model system for removing neuroblastoma cells from bone marrow using monoclonal antibodies and magnetic immunobeads. Cancer Res 1986; 46:846-851.

6. Kamby C, Vejborg I, Daugaard S, Guldhammer B, Dirksen H, Rossing N, Mouridsen HT: Clinical and radiologic characteristics of bone metastases in breast cancer. Cancer 1987; 60:2524-2531.

7. Morecki S, Pavlotsky S, Margel S, Slavin S. Purging breast cancer cells in preparation for autologous bone marrow transplantation. Bone Marrow Transplant 1987 1:357-363.

8. Tondini C, Pap SA, Hayes DF, Elias AD, Kufe DW: Evaluation of monoclonal antibody DF3 conjugated with Ricin as a specific immunotoxin for in vitro purging of human bone marrow. Cancer Research 1990; 50:1170-1175.

9. Frankel AE, Ring DB, Tringale F, Hsieh-Ma ST: Tissue distribution of breast cancer-associated antigens defined by monoclonal antibodies. J Biol Response Mod 1985, 4:273-286.

10. Shpall E, Jones R, Bast R, Shogan J, Ross M, Edwards S, Eggleston S, Johnston C, Affronti M, Coniglio D, Peters W: 4-hydroperoxy-cyclophosphamide (4-HC) of breast cancer from the ficolled mono-nuclear cell fraction (FMNCF) of bone marrow. Proc Am Soc Clin Oncol 1989; 8:42.

11. Shpall EJ, Bast RC Jr, Joines WT, Jones RB, Anderson I, Johnston C, Eggleston S, Tepperberg M, Edwards S, Peters WP: Immunomagnetic purging of breast cancer from bone marrow for autologous transplantation: Bone Marrow Transplantation 1991; 7:145-151.

12. Meropol NJ, Overmoyer BA, Stadtmauer EA, Lazarus HM, Williams SF: High-dose chemotherapy with autologous stem cell support for breast cancer. Oncology 1992; 6:53-69.

13. Jereb B, Bretsky SS, Vogel R. Helson L: Age and prognosis in neuroblas-

toma: review of 112 patients younger than 2 years. Am J Pediatr Hematol Oncol 1984, 6:233-243.

14. Hartmann O, Kalifa C, Benhamou E, Patte C, Flamant F, Jullien C, Beaujean F, Lemerle J: Treatment of advanced neuroblastoma with high-dose melphalan and autologous bone marrow transplantation. Cancer Chemother Pharmacol 1986; 16:165-169.

15. August CA, Serota FT, Koch PA, Burkey E, Schlesinger H, Elkins WL, Evans AE, D'Angio GJ: Treatment of advanced neuroblastoma with supralethal chemotherapy, radiation, and allogeneic or autologous marrow reconstitution. J Clin Oncol, 1984, 2:609-616.

16. Pole JG, Casper J, Elfenbein G, Gee A, Gross S, Janssen W, Koch P, Marcus R, Pick T, Shuster J, Spruce W, Thomas P, Yeager A: High-dose chemo-radiotherapy supported by marrow infusions for advanced neuroblastoma: A pediatric oncology group study. J Clin Oncol 1991; 9:152-158.

17. Kushner BH, Gulati SC, Kwon J-H, O'Reilly RJ, Exelby PR, Cheung N-KV. High-Dose Melphalan With 6-Hydroxydopamine-Purged Autologous Bone Marrow Transplantation for Poor-Risk Neuroblastoma. Cancer 1991, 68:242-247.

18. Gulati, SC, Kwon, J-H, Kushner BH, Cheung N-K, Atzpodien J, Shum K, Clarkson BD. In Vitro Chemopurification of Neuroblastoma Cells: Comparison of 6-Hydroxydopamine and Ascorbic Acid with 4-Hydroperoxycyclophosphamide. Cancer Investigation 1989; 7:417-422.

19. Kushner BH, O'Reilly RJ, Mandell LR, Gulati SC, LaQuaglia M, Cheung N-KV: Myeloablative Combination Chemotherapy Without Total Body Irradiation for Neuroblastoma. J Clin Oncol, 1991, 9:274-279.

20. Treleaven JG, Ugelstad J, Philip T, Gibson FM, Rembaum A, Caine GD, Kemshead JT: Removal of neuroblastoma cells from bone marrow with mono-clonal antibodies conjugated to magnetic microspheres. Lancet 1984, 1:70-75.

21. Kemshead JT, Heath L, Gibson FM, Katz F, Richmond F, Treleaven JG, Ugelstad J: Magnetic microspheres and monoclonal antibodies for the depletion of neuroblastoma cells from bone marrow: experiences, improvements and observations. Br J Cancer 1986, 54:771-778.

22. Philip T, Bernard JL, Zucker JM, Pinkerton R, Lutz P, Bordigoni P, Plouvier E, Robert A, Carton R, Philippe N, Philip I, Chauvin F, Favrot M: High-dose chemoradiotherapy with bone marrow transplantation as consolidation treatment in neuroblastoma: An unselected group of stage IV patients over 1 year of age. J Clin Oncol, 1987 5:266-271.

23. Hartmann O, Benhamou E, Beaujean F, Kalifa C, Lejars O, Patte C, Behard C, Flamant F, Thyss A, Deville A, Vannier JP, Pautard-Muchemble B, Lemerle J: Repeated high-dose chemotherapy followed by purged autologous bone marrow transplantation as consolidation therapy in metastatic neuroblastoma. J Clin Oncol, 1987, 5:1205-1211.

24. Atzpodien J, Gulati SC, Kwon JH, Kushner BH, Schimazaki C, Buhrer C, Oz S, Kolitz JE, Welte K, Clarkson BD. Anti-Tumor Efficacy of Interleukin-2-Activated Killer Cells in Human Neuroblastoma ex vivo. Expl Cell Biol 1988, 56:236-244.

25. Rosen G, Juergens H, Caparros B, Nirenberg A, Huvos AG, Marcove

RC: Combination chemotherapy (T-6) in the multidisciplinary treatment of Ewing's sarcoma. Natl Cancer Inst Monogr 1981, 56:289-299.

26. Wilkins RM, Pritchard DJ, Burgert EO Jr, Unni KK: Ewing's sarcoma of bone: Experience with 140 patients. Cancer 1986, 58:2551-2555.

27. Cornbleet MA, Corringham RET, Prentice HG: Treatment of Ewing's sarcoma with high-dose melphalan and autologous bone marrow transplantation. Cancer Treat Rep 1981, 65:241-244.

28. Jacobsen AB, Wist EA, Solheim P: Treatment of Ewing's sarcoma with high-dose melphalan and autologous bone marrow rescue. In: Autologous Bone Marrow Transplantation and Solid Tumors. Edited by G McVie, O Dalesio, EI Smith. New York, Raven Press, 1984, 157-160.

29. Gulati SC, Kwon J-H, Atzpodien J, Triche TJ, Colvin OM, Clarkson BD: In vitro chemosensitivity of two Ewing's sarcoma cell lines: Implication for autologous bone marrow transplantation. Can Invest 1989; 7:411-416.

30. Atzpodien J, Gulati SC, Schimazaki C, Buhrer C, Oz S, Kwon JH, Kolitz JE, Clarkson BD. Ewing's Sarcoma: ex vivo sensitivity towards natural and lymphokine-activated killing. Oncology 1988, 45:437-443.

31. Stahel RA, Mabry M, Skarin AT, Speak J, Bernal SD. Detection of bone marrow metastasis in small-cell lung cancer by monoclonal antibody. J Clin. Oncol 1985, 3:455-461.

32. Vredenburgh JJ, Ball ED: Elimination of small cell carcinoma of the lung from human bone marrow by monoclonal antibodies and immunomagnetic beads. Cancer Research 1990, 50:7216-7220.

33. Meagher R, Rothman S, Paul S, Koberna P, Wilmer C, Baucco P: Purging of small cell lung cancer cells using ethiotos (WR 2721) and light activated merocyanine 540 phototreatment. Cancer Res 1989, 49:3637-3641.

CHAPTER 6

DETECTION AND SIGNIFICANCE OF MINIMAL RESIDUAL DISEASE

Recurrence of disease is the most common complication of autologous stem cell transplant.[1-4] Most likely the relapse is due to the growth of minimal residual disease (MRD) in the patient either due to incomplete eradication in vivo or due to the infusion of cancer cells with the stem cell rescue. In allogeneic BMT, small amounts of infused lymphocytes present in the bone marrow harvest cause additional complications of graft-versus-host disease and if these lymphocytes are purged, the risk of graft rejection is increased.[5-7] Recent investigations have clearly shown the persistence of host cells (mixed chimerism) after allogeneic BMT in some of the patients.[8-10] The long-term significance of this mixed chimeric state is now being evaluated. It appears that long-term persistence of host cells correlates with relapse. Improving methods to quantitate MRD will provide more reliable data to properly define the significance of MRD in the hematopoietic stem cells being infused into the patient. Furthermore, such techniques will also be useful in deciding the in vivo elimination of cancer. The likely causes of relapse in patients undergoing transplantation are due to multiple factors, some of them are detailed in other parts of this book. The relapse can occur from: (1) ineffective treatment of the patient; and (2) infusion of cancer cells at stem cell transplantation (ineffective purging).

Several methods are available to quantitate cancer cells contaminating the normal hematopoietic elements in the bone marrow and the techniques were discussed in the previous chapters and are briefly summarized in Table 1.[1-4] Standard morphological analysis is usually not accurate below 5% (exceptions would be observing an Auer rod in a patient with acute non-lymphoblastic leukemia or finding a cluster of malignant cells in a patient with breast cancer). Considering that most investigators infuse 10 billion cells at transplantation, a contamination of up to 100 million cancer cells can then be infused into the patient with significant theoretical risk of relapse.[2,3] The clonal defects in T- and B-lymphocytes have been utilized for fluorescence-activated cell sorting analysis or immunoperoxidase stains. Cytogenetics is specific for only a few diseases and is too labor intensive to have any significant role in detecting MRD at this time. Improvements in instruments may change the role of cytogenetic analysis. Preferential culture of malignant cell requires technical expertise, does not work for many diseases and is not reproducible.[12,13]

Table 1. Methods used for the detection of minimal residual cancer in the bone marrow

Method	% Usual Sensitivity	Problem
Morphology	1 to 5	Not reliable
Phenotypic Markers (FACS, immunoperoxidase stains)	1 to 5	Usually not reliable
Cytogenetics	1 to 2	Labor intensive
Genotypic Markers		Not seen frequently
Aneuploidy, Hyperploidy, etc. by cytometry	0.01 to 0.001	
Genetic Defect (PCR, FISH)	0.001 to 0.0001	High false positive and negatives;
Preferential Culture of Cancer Cells	0.01 to 0.001	Occasional success

Analysis of aneuploid or hyperdiploid cells by flow-cytometer is only applicable to an occasional patient. Recent studies suggest that polymerase chain reaction (PCR) is the most sensitive approach for detection of MRD.[3,4,14-17] The PCR is a specific enzyme-related technique (currently employing DNA polymerase from thermophylic bacterium is utilized) that amplifies signals attached to target piece of DNA.[18] The sequence at the ends of this target must be known to chemically synthesize oligonucleotide primers that are identical to the 5' ends of the double stranded target DNA sequence (the DNA strands are anti-parallel, therefore these two ends will be at opposite ends of the target, and on opposite strands). The target DNA is then mixed with both primers, the four nucleotide triphosphates (dATP, dGTP, dCTP, and dTTP), a magnesium containing buffer, and a heat-stable DNA polymerase. The mixture is then heated to 94°C, which denatures the DNA and this separates the DNA into single strands. Upon cooling the mix to a temperature just below the melting temperature of the primer/DNA duplex (usually between 55°C and 65°C), the primers will anneal to their complementary regions. These oligonucleotides will now serve as primers for DNA polymerase-directed synthesis of new DNA, which is identical to the target strand. Thus, the DNA has now been duplicated in the region between the two primers. If this mix is again cycled through denaturation, annealing, and synthesis, a four-fold increase in target DNA is anticipated. Further cycles lead to significant amplification of the DNA, so that after 20 cycles, approximately one million fold amplification may occur. The amplified signal can be analyzed by various methods. For example, Southern Blot analysis detects 0.1 pg of DNA or by ultraviolet visualization of ethidium bromide stain which usually detects 10 ng of DNA.[14]

In a new approach, to further enhance the signal, a second round of PCR amplification is carried out using "nested" primers (after the first round of amplification is performed as detailed above).[14] The nested primer falls a few nucleotides within the primers used in the first PCR and, therefore allow further amplification of the target sequence. This approach is particularly useful when the initial PCR is difficult to interpret. The sensitivity of PCR in detecting a small amount of target DNA is unfortunately associated with the problem of false positive results. Extreme precautions in the laboratory are needed to avoid such problems and to obtain meaningful results.[3,14] Another shortcoming of the PCR is the relative lack of quantitation. This is especially true when the tumor samples that have chromosomal translocations are used. In such situations, it is often difficult to accurately detect the amount of tumor cell involvement. A semiquantitative estimation can usually be made based upon the intensity of the bands as compared to known contaminated samples. However, reverse PCR, where RNA is used instead of DNA for the reaction is even more difficult to quantitate. Another approach includes the use of competitive PCR where a primer is constructed with a similar sequence to that which is to be amplified, for example, of the bcr-abl breakpoint and such primer is then used to construct a megaprimer, which can then be added to the PCR reaction to quantitate the amount.[14] Another quantitation approach using the CDR III PCR has been developed whereby material is cloned into phage and a quantitative estimate of the tumor-involved sequences is compared to normal uninvolved sequences. These approaches may become useful in following patients with respect to their disease status after treatment.[3,17]

PCR technology is particularly useful in clinical situations where a translocation has occurred and resulted in hybrid gene, i.e., bcr-abl product. The resultant hybrid gene gets its terminal parts from two different genes. The oligonucleotide primers are therefore unique and produce an exponential expansion of the translocated gene. In contrast, if the gene is not translocated, the amplification using these unique primers will merely be arithmetic.[3,14,16] Analyses described above have been extremely valuable in patients with known chromosomal translocations such as the t(14:18) chromosomal translocation of non-Hodgkin's lymphoma, the t(9:22) chromosomal translocation found in the majority of patients with chronic myeloid leukemia (CML), and for a significant proportion of patients with acute lymphoblastic leukemia (ALL).[19,20] The use of PCR has also been expanded to acute promyelocytic leukemias with t(15:17) translocations.[21] More generic approaches, for example in patients with T-cell receptor rearrangement related lymphoma or leukemia are also available for a small number of patients.[17]

EVALUATING MRD AFTER CHEMOTHERAPY

Recurrence of any malignancy after achieving remission supports the concept that MRD was present. Detecting MRD is often difficult. In one study, PCR-based approaches were used to study childhood ALL. Using CDR III PCR, a quantitative assessment of MRD was made (limit of sensitivity being one tumor cell in 10^5 normal cells). Marrow samples were evaluated by PCR following standard induction chemotherapy. A 3- to 4-log reduction in the number of leukemic cells were found in those patients who entered clinical remission.[17] Eight patients were examined further. In four of these patients, residual disease was detected in at least one follow-up bone marrow sample taken while in remission. A dramatic rise in the number of leukemic cells was found three months prior to clinical relapse in one patient. Other studies find similar approaches useful for managing patients with T-cell lymphomas.

EVALUATING MRD AFTER PURGING

PCR technology has been most useful in detecting tumor cells (only if a PCR recognizable signal is known to be present prior to purging, only few diseases are known to have such specific defects at this time) before and after purging of the bone marrow. In ex vivo experiments, the PCR assay was found to be equivalent to the clonogenic assay. The most dramatic proof of the effectiveness of purging was also discussed in Chapter 1. Among the 114 patients with known BCL-2 positive disease, the bone marrow was evaluated for presence or absence of BCL-2 before and after purging. Ex vivo therapy utilized one to three antibodies (specific to the patient's lymphoma cells) with complement. This therapy eradicated BCL-2 positivity in 57 patients. Relapse of the disease in the patient was correlated with respect to BCL-2 and is presented in Table 2.[4] Even though the follow-up is short and more patients are expected to relapse, a conservative estimate is made of false positives and negatives. From the data presented, one can postulate that other mechanisms are also involved in predicting the success or failure of AUSCT in patients with lymphoma. So far, only 67% of the patients who were infused with

Table 2. Clinical course of 114 patients with BCL-2 positive lymphoma, purged with antibodies, evaluated again

BM involved	BCL-2 by PCR (subsequent relapse)		Total # of PTs
	Negative	Positive	
no	35 (1)	30 (10)	65
<5%	20 (2)	18 (10)	38
>5%	2 (1)	9 (6)	11
Total	57 (4)	57 (26)	114

"True negative" BCL-2 negative, normal morphology; Correlation with no subsequent relapse	52/55 = 95%*
BCL-2 positive, BM involvement; with subsequent relapse	6/9 = 67%*
BCL-2 and morphology negative with subsequent relapse	3/55 = 5%*
BCL-2 positive (morphology negative), subsequently no relapse	28/48 = 58%*

*Short follow up. Data abstracted from reference #4

BCL-2 positive cells have relapsed. It is possible that some of the other 33% of the patients will eventually relapse, or if no relapse occurs, one can assume that the body may clear the disease by other mechanisms, i.e., immunomodulatory, or that the BCL-2 positivity was due to the presence of inactive cells. The 5% false negative results observed so far may be due to the inability to diagnose the BCL-2 signal or could also be due to relapse from other mechanism, i.e., drug resistance, p53 alterations etc. Furthermore, the study found that the most important predictor of continued clinical remission was the achievement of PCR negativity after purging, thus proving that purging conditions utilized were effective. Another unsolved issue is that relapses occurred mainly in the area of previous disease, which may suggest that the conditioning regimen of the patient was inadequate and plays an important role in the overall success of purged AUSCT.[4]

In the recent review of European experience in patients with acute nonlymphoblastic leukemia (AML), it was observed that purging bone marrow with mafosfamide was mainly helpful to patients receiving TBI containing conditioning regimen.[22] The data is summarized in Table 3. Improved strategies need to be developed for treating and monitoring patients with AML, especially in second and third remission.

MRD IN PERIPHERAL BLOOD

Enthusiasm has now developed for improving the quality of peripheral blood stem cells (PBSC) harvested for transplantation, as the engraftment especially of megakaryocytic series after PBSCT is abrupt.[23,24] There is significant interest in properly quantitating the MRD in PBSC. Unfortunately, even though the presence of MRD is usually found in PBSC for patients with lymphoma and leukemia, it is not possible to properly quantitate it. Therefore, all of the issues regarding possible involvement of bone marrow as detailed in this chapter are also relevant to the study of PBSC transplantation.[3,25-29] The possibility of higher relapse rate with PBSCT when compared to no stem cell rescue should be considered against the short-term benefit of early hematopoietic reconstitution. This issue is often not addressed in publications.

MRD IN ALLOGENEIC BMT

Evaluation of bcr-abl gene after allogeneic BMT has shown positive signals even when the Ph chromosome is negative. The long-term implications require a better understanding of MRD. A recent report describes persistence of bcr-abl gene in some patients (Figure 1) with CML after allogenic BMT.[10]

As better methods for detecting MRD are developed,[3,30,31] especially the ability to detect genetic abnormalities in single cells with fluorescence in situ hybridization, we may be able to better define the best method of purging and subsequently prove the clinical benefit of transplantation by using purged hematopoietic stem cells.

Table 3. Prognostic factors in predicting clinical benefit of mafosfamide purging in AML receiving TBI as part of conditioning regimen

Group	Prognostic variable AML first remission	% Disease-free survival			Most likely explanation
		Purged	Unpurged	△ Benefit	
1A	Remission to AUBMT < 6 mo	65	45	20	Leukemic burden is treatable (partial?) By mafosfamide purging
1B	Remission to AUBMT > 6 mo	58	58	0	Leukemic regrowth in-vivo, drug resistance, develop new strategies
	AML first remission				
2A	DX to remission < 40 days	62	65	-3	Low leukemia burden after induction, purge not beneficial
2B	DX to remission > 40 days	63	41	22	residual leukemia, in vivo and in BM harvest, partially treatable with mafosfamide purge
		% relapse rate			
		Purged	Unpurged	△ Benefit	
	AML second remission				
3A	HSC harvest 1st remission	36	68	32	Mafosfamide purging helpful, significant leukemia in vivo
3B	HSC harvest 2nd remission	64	52	-12	Mafosfamide purging not useful. High leukemia burden. Drug resistance. Need new strategies

Data abstracted from figures published by Labopin and Gorin. Leukemia 6: Suppl 4; 95-99, 1992.

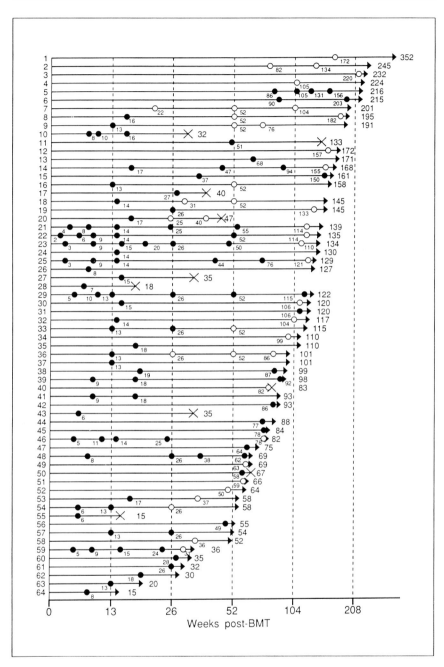

Figure 1. Clinical course of 64 patients with CML after allogeneic BMT. Samples were analyzed for the presence of bcr-abl gene by polymerase chain reaction. Closed circles were positive for the bcr-abl signal, open circles were negative for bcr-abl signal. Arrow at the right side donates patients who are alive at last follow up; and x on the right side donates patients who died (weeks after BMT). Reproduced with permission.[10]

REFERENCES

1. Gross S, Gee AP, Worthington-White DA, eds: Progress in clinical and biological research, bone marrow purging and processing. Vol 333 Alan R. Liss Publisher, 1990.

2. Gulati SC, Lemoli RM, Acaba L, Igarashi T, Wasserheit C, Mustafa F: Purging in autologous and allogeneic bone marrow transplantation. Current Opinion in Oncology 1992, 4:264-271.

3. Negrin RS: Use of the polymerase chain reaction for the detection of tumor cell involvement of bone marrow and peripheral blood: Implications for purging. J Hematotherapy 1992; 1:361-368.

4. Gribben JG, Freedman AS, Neuberg D, Roy DC, Blake KW, Woo SD, Grossbarb ML, Rabinowe SN, Coral F, Freeman GJ, Ritz J, Nadler LM: Immunologic purging of marrow assessed by PCR before autologous bone marrow transplantation for B-cell lymphoma. New England Journal of Medicine 1991; 325:1525-1533.

5. Frame JN, Collins NH, Cartagena T, Waldman H, O'Reilly RJ, Dupont B, Kernan NA: T cell depletion of human bone marrow: comparison of Campath-1 plus complement, anti-T-cell ricin A chain immunotoxin and soybean agglutinin alone or in combination with sheep erythrocytes or immunomagnetic beads. Transplantation 1989; 47:984-988.

6. Keever CA, Small TN, Flomenberg N, Heller G, Pekle K, Black P, Pecora A, Gilio A, Kernan N, O'Reilly RJ: Immune reconstitution following bone marrow transplantation: comparison of recipients of T cell depleted marrow with recipients of conventional marrow grafts. Blood 1989; 73:1340-1350.

7. Roux E, Abdi K, Speiser D, Helg C, Chapuis B, Jeannet M, Roosnek E: Characterization of mixed chimerism in patients with chronic myeloid leukemia transplanted with T-cell-depleted bone marrow: Involvement of different hematologic lineages before and after relapse. Blood 1993; 81:243-248.

8. McGlave P, Bartsch G, Anasetti C, Ash R, Beatty P, Gajewski J, Kernan NA: Unrelated donor marrow transplantation therapy for chronic myelogenous leukemia: Initial experience of the National Marrow Donor Program. Blood 1993; 81:543-550.

9. Cunningham I, Castro-Malaspina H, Flomenberg N, Gulati SC, Shank B, Collins N, Keever C, O'Reilly RJ: Improved results of bone marrow transplantation for chronic myelogenous leukemia using marrow depleted of T-cells by soybean lectin agglutination and E-rosette depletion. Progress in Bone Marrow Transplantation Alan R. Liss, Inc. 1987; 359-363.

10. Miyamura K, Tahara T, Tanimoto M, Morishita Y, Kawashima K, Morishima Y, Saito H, Tsuzuki S, Takeyama K, Kodera Y, Matsuyama K, Hirabayashi N, Yamada H, Naito K, Imai K, Sakamaki H, Asai O, Mizutani S: Long persistent bcr-abl positive transcript detected by polymerase chain reaction after marrow transplant for chronic myelogenous leukemia without clinical relapse: A study of 64 patients. Blood 1993; 81:1089-1093.

11. Cartun RW, Pedersen CA: An immunocytochemical technique offering increased sensitivity and a lowered cost with a streptavidin horseradish-peroxidase conjugate. J Histotech 1989; 12:273.

12. Estrov Z, Grunberger T, Dube ID, Wang YP, Freedman MH: Detection of residual acute lymphoblastic leukemia cells in cultures of bone marrow obtained during remission. N Engl J Med 1986; 315:538-542.

13. Miller CB, Zehnbauer BA, Piantadosi S, Rowley SD, Jones RJ: Correlation of occult clonogenic leukemia drug sensitivity with relapse after autologous bone marrow transplantation. Blood 1991; 78:1125-1131.

14. Hooberman AL: The use of the polymerase chain reaction in clinical oncology. Oncology 1992; 6:25-36.

15. Lee M-S, Chang KS, Cabanillas F, Freireich EJ, Trujillo JM, Stass SA: Detection of minimal residual cells carrying the t(14;18) by DNA sequence amplification. Science 1987; 175-178.

16. Negrin RS, Blume KG: The use of the polymerase chain reaction for the detection of minimal residual malignant disease. Blood 1991; 78:255-258.

17. Yamada M, Wasserman R, Lange B, Reichard BA, Womer RB, Rovera G: Minimal residual disease in childhood B-lineage lymphoblastic leukemia. The New England Journal of Medicine 1990; 323:448-455.

18. Saiki RK, Gelfand DH, Stoffel S, Scharf SJ, Higuchi R, Horn GT, Mullis KB, Erlich HA: Primer-directed enzymatic amplification of DNA with a thermostable DNA polymerase. Science 239:487-491.

19. Cresenzi M, Seto M, Herzig GP, Weiss PD, Griffith RC, Korsmeyer JC: Thermostable DNA polymerase chain amplification of t(14;18) chromosomal breakpoints and detection of minimal residual disease. Proc Natl Acad Sci 1988, 85:4869-4873.

20. Stetler-Stevenson M, Raffeld M, Cohen P, Cossman J: Detection of occult follicular lymphoma by specific DNA amplification. Blood 1988; 72:1822-1825.

21. Biondi A, Rambaldi A, Pandolfi PP, Rossi V, Giudici G, Alcalay M, Lo Coco F, Diverio D, Pogliani EM, Lanzi EM, Mandelli F, Masera G, Barbui T, Pelicci PG: Molecular monitoring of the myl/retinoic acid receptor-α fusion gene in acute promyelocytic leukemia by polymerase chain reaction. Blood 1992; 80:492-497.

22. Labopin M, Gorin NC: Autologous bone marrow transplantation in 2502 patients with acute leukemia in Europe: a retrospective study. Leukemia 1992; 6(Suppl 4):95-99.

23. Gianni AM, Bregni M, Stern AC, Siena S, Tarella C, Pileri A, Bonadonna G: Granulocyte-macrophage colony-stimulating factor to harvest circulating haemopoietic stem cells for autotransplantation. Lancet 1989; 580-585.

24. Sheridan WP, Begley CG, Juttner CA, Szer J, Bikto L, Maher D, McGrath K, Morstyn G, Fox R: Effect of peripheral blood progenitor cells mobilized by filgrastim (G-CSF) on platelet recovery after high-dose chemotherapy. Lancet 1992; 339:640-644.

25. Horning SJ, Galili N, Cleary M, Sklar J: Detection of non-Hodgkin's lymphoma in the peripheral blood by analysis of antigen receptor gene rearrangements: Results of a prospective study. Blood 1990; 75:1139-1145.

26. Miller WH Jr, Kakizuka A, Frankel SR, Warrell RP Jr, DeBlasio A, Kristi L, Evans RM, Dmitrovsky E: Reverse transcription polymerase chain reaction for the rearranged retinoic acid receptor α clarifies diagnosis and

detects minimal residual disease in acute promyelocytic leukemia. Proc Natl Acad Sci 1992; 89:2694-2698.

27. Negrin RS, Pesando J, Long GD, Chao NJ, Horning SJ, Blume KG: Comparison of tumor cell contamination of purged bone marrow to peripheral blood mononuclear cells assessed by PCR in non-Hodgkin's lymphoma. Blood 1992; 80(suppl 1):931.

28. Moss TJ, Xu Z-J, Mansour VH, Hardwick A, Kulcinski D, Ishizawa L, Law P, Gee A: Quantitation of tumor cell removal from bone marrow: A preclinical model. J of Hematotherapy 1992; 1:65-73.

29. Billadeau D, Quam L, Thomas W, Kay N, Greipp P, Kyle R, Oken MM, VanNess B: Detection and quantitation of malignant cells in the peripheral blood of multiple myeloma patients. Blood 1992; 80:1818-1824.

30. Zelenetz AD, Chu G, Galili N, Bangs CD, Horning SJ, Donlon TA, Cleary ML, Levy R. Enhanced detection of the t(14;18) translocation in malignant lymphoma using pulsed-field gel electrophosphoresis. Blood 1991; 78:1552-1560.

31. Tkachuk DC, Westbrook CA, Andreeff M, Donlon TA, Cleary ML, Suryanarayan K, Homge M, Redner A, Gray J, Pinkel D: Detection of bcr-abl fusion in chronic myelogeneous leukemia by in situ hybridization. Science 1990; 250:559-562.

CHAPTER 7

HEMATOPOIETIC ENGRAFTMENT AND ROLE OF GROWTH FACTORS

The quality and speed of hematopoietic recovery after intermediate and high dose chemotherapy has become the subject of intense investigations in the past few years.[1-7] Significant research has been performed to prove that various methods (GM-CSF, G-CSF, primed or unprimed peripheral blood stem cells used alone or in combination with bone marrow) can cause faster hematopoietic recovery and thus save hospitalization costs.[8-19] We still need to learn more about the quality of hematopoietic engraftment and the risk of such therapies especially to prove that such manipulations (including various methods of purging) do not alter the relapse rate or cause patients to develop secondary malignancies or late complications of graft failure.[2,20] The situation is even more difficult for patients undergoing allogeneic BMT because immunomodulatory dysfunction can further cause problems with the hematopoietic system (Figure 1).[2,7,14] In this regard, the higher incidence of CMV infection in patients receiving allogeneic BMT can delay hematopoietic engraftment.[21,22] Quantitation of CFU-GM used to be the best predictor of hematopoietic engraftment, but several issues have now complicated the correlation. Specifically, CFU-GM assay is not standardized from institution to institution. It only measures one or a few limited types of already committed hematopoietic progenitors, it does not predict the time to engraftment in all situations and it requires 10-14 days to obtain results.[6,17,23]

Another assay based on the presence CD-34 antigen on early hematopoietic progenitor evaluates the hematopoietic progenitor pool in a matter of hours. This assay can be easily standardized from institution to institution.[5-7] Unfortunately CD-34 assays are hard to perform on frozen thawed cells.

Several groups have examined the correlation between CD-34 infused cells and engraftment and have found that it is predictive of the number of CFU-GM colonies. These colonies may be found in peripheral blood leukocytes collected following stem cell mobilization by chemotherapy. In one recent analysis,[6] it appears that a positive correlation exists between CD-34+ cell fraction and CFU-GM colony formation in peripheral blood from normal individuals, or from individuals recovering from cyclophosphamide chemotherapy and receiving no concomitant leukocyte stimulation therapy. Poor correlation was observed when similar data from bone marrow trans-

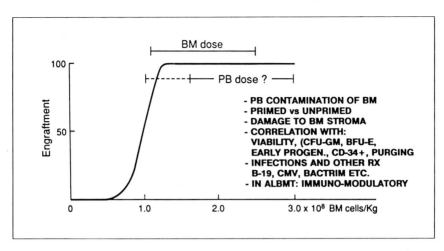

Figure 1. Some of the factors which influence the quality of engraftment. The engraftment can be further subclassified: 1) speed of engraftment of each lineage; 2) reestablishment of all hemopoietic lineages, i.e., engraftment of red cells, white cells and megakaryocyte series; 3) higher risk of relapse when a larger dose of cells is infused should also be considered; and 4) effect of other factors, some of which are detailed in this figure.

plantation was analyzed. Accordingly, application of this assay as a substitute for the CFU-GM assay needs further investigations. The authors advocate adoption of this assay as a parallel to the CFU-GM, in that it may yield complimentary information and it does retain the advantages of rapid result and ease of standardization. Patients with AML tend to have the slowest hematopoietic engraftment after AUBMT. Some of the factors which influence hematopoietic reconstitution are listed below:[2,17,18,20-27]

1) Effect of primary disease and its treatment on subsequent engraftment
2) Acute residual toxicity of therapy before bone marrow harvest
3) Quality and quantity of bone marrow harvested, cell number, viability, CFU-GM, and BFU-E dose
4) Effect of bone marrow purging, processing, storage, thawing and infusion
5) Effect of bone marrow cryopreservation, which may even be different for malignant cells when compared with normal hematopoietic cells.
6) Microenvironment conditions during the time of early transplant, i.e., effect of various infections (especially B19 parvovirus, cytomegalovirus, Epstein-Barr virus, and other viruses), various drugs (especially antibiotic), vitamin levels, and release of various growth factors from the microenvironment and host cells.
7) In patients undergoing allogeneic BMT; additional factors include: GVHD, treatment of GVHD, genetic disparity (nonmajor HLA type), and immunosurveillance dysfunction.

Other factors that affect the rate of engraftment need to be considered. The use of drugs during transplant, such as trimethroprim-sulfamethoxazole and acyclovir, have been considered as possible cause of delay in engraftment. Correlation of in vitro assays with engraftment has been attempted. Among the most frequently used are progenitor assays where aliquots of either the fresh or cryopreserved bone marrow are plated and the amounts of myeloid progenitors (CFU-GM) and erythroid progenitors (BFU-E) are determined. Quantification of early progenitor cells (CD-34+) is also being explored. From the theoretical benefit of the methods described above, the data suggests that CD-34 positivity is probably the most reliable predictor of engraftment when PBSC from previously untreated patients are utilized, but the disagreement persists as to the true benefit of the assay, especially in heavily pretreated patients.[5-7,17,18,23] The correlation of CD-34 positivity in bone marrow and subsequent engraftment is not as good as that with PBSCT.[6]

In a recent review of published literature,[17,23] the dosage of PBSC necessary for hematologic recovery was provided. Although similar doses of MNCs were used, the reviewer found a striking variation of the dosage of CFU-GM infused between centers which was certainly related to the differences in the performance of the colony assay. In spite of the variation in estimating dosage, rapid engraftment was observed in nearly all of the studies reviewed. Efforts to enhance the formation of colonies using synergistic recombinant growth factors will likely improve the reproducibility of this assay. The most promising laboratory method currently available is the measurement of CD-34+ cells by flow cytometry. Standardization of the preparation and analysis of cells will help establish the value of this measurement. Finally, analysis of the data from three centers where dosage of PBSC was compared to hematologic recovery revealed variations in patient populations, mobilization protocols and the high-dose chemotherapy used. Correlation between CFU-GM dose and the rate of hematopoietic reconstitution was usually observed. Multivariate analysis of 65 patients transplanted with either allogeneic (n = 14) or autologous (n = 13) bone marrow or chemotherapy mobilized PBSC (n = 38) showed that the CFU-GM dose is the only independent variable influencing neutrophil or platelet reconstitution. A further analysis of these data revealed that a threshold effect exists, i.e., an optimal number of CFU-GM is required to ensure rapid hematopoietic reconstitution. These data suggest an optimum number of 20-50 x 10^4 CFU-GM/kg body weight (BW) which is consistent with two previous reports. Likewise, 2 x 10^6 CD-34+ cells/kg BW represent conservative doses that usually result in rapid recovery of neutrophils and platelets. Lower doses of 5-20 x 10^4 CFU-GM and 0.5-2 x 10^6 CD-34+ cells/kg BW may represent threshold or minimal doses that provide sustained engraftment; however, further experience will be required to establish these doses as safe for engraftment. Differences in cell preparations obtained using different mobilization protocols will initially necessitate the evaluation of the effect of drug(s) on hematopoietic stem cell harvest and subsequent engraftment for each variation in the protocol. Experiments in mice have shown that there is a minimum number of approximately 5,000 untreated cells [corresponding to one or two CFU-GM or spleen colonies (CFU-S)] which if transplanted, allow survival of lethally irradiated mice. There also exists a maximum value for the number of hematopoietic progenitors in a marrow graft, i.e., no significant increase in the hematopoietic engraftment is noted when over 5 million cells are used for transplant. The presence of this maximum value for transplanted progenitors and variations in culture techniques is probably the reason why previous studies have not always shown a correlation between CFU-GM content and hematologic recovery after bone marrow transplantation.[17]

HEMATOPOIETIC GROWTH FACTORS AND ENGRAFTMENT

The clinical benefit of GM-CSF and G-CSF was established early in patients undergoing autologous BMT. Several trials now support the use of GM-CSF and G-CSF to decrease the duration of neutropenia and associated cost of hospitalization. Availability of growth factors to prime the harvest of PBSC has decreased neutropenia and has also reduced the number of platelet transfusions and days with thrombocytopenia in patients undergoing high dose therapy.[5-15]

As mentioned before, in patients undergoing allogeneic BMT, other immunomodulatory factors and prophylactic treatment of GVH with methotrexate, cyclosporine, etc. can effect the hematopoietic engraftment rate. Recent data suggests that growth factors also benefit patients undergoing allogeneic BMT.[8-11]

In a prospective randomized study, five European transplant centers compared recombinant human granulocyte-macrophage colony-stimulating factor (rhGM-CSF; mammalian glycosylated) with a placebo in patients undergoing allogeneic T-cell-depleted BMT.[10] GM-CSF was administered in a dose of 8 μg glycoprotein (5.5 μ protein)/kg/d, as a continuous intravenous (IV) infusion for 14 days, starting 3 hours after bone marrow infusion. Fifty-seven patients entered and completed the study. Median age of the recipients was 34 years (range, 17 to 51 y). All donors were HLA-identical, MLC-nonreactive siblings. Marrow grafts were depleted of T lymphocytes either by counterflow centrifugation (n = 42) or by immunological methods (n = 15). Twenty-nine patients received GM-CSF and 28 patients received the placebo. The leukocyte count and the absolute neutrophil count were significantly higher in the GM-CSF-treated group from day +9 to day +14 after bone marrow transplantation (BMT). This was also true for the monocyte count from day +12 to day +21. Also, neutrophil (>0.1 and >0.3 x 10^9/L) and leukocyte (>0.3 and >0.5 x 10^9/L) recovery was significantly faster for the patients given GM-CSF. The incidence of graft-versus-host disease (GVHD) and transplant-related mortality were not different in both groups. However, the number of bronchopneumonias was significantly lower in the rhGM-CSF treated group (P = .03). Long-term follow-up showed a trend to better overall disease-free survival at two years and a trend to a lower relapse risk in patients treated with GM-CSF. In this study, GM-CSF significantly increased neutrophil and monocyte counts after BMT. This resulted in a decreased number of pneumonias, without an increase in incidence of GVHD or relapse.

There is a large variation in the dose and route of administration of the growth factors in various studies. Some of the side effects can decrease if lower dosages are used and/or if the therapy is given over a prolonged period. A subcutaneous schedule on a twice daily basis needs to be explored for proving clinical benefit as it is easy to perform as an out-patient or in-patient basis and can usually be done without major medical supervision.

High dose cytotoxic therapy results in drop of the neutrophil count to zero, and often the time required to reach the neutrophil count of 500 or 1,000 per cubic millimeter after stem cell infusion (or last day of chemotherapy) is used as an index of the risk of infection. Similarly the number of days for platelet counts to recover over 50,000 or 100,000 per cubic millimeter and total units of platelets and/or packed red cell transfusion and/or improvement in the reticulocyte count is used as an index of hematopoietic recovery. Even though a true correlation of the factors mentioned above with clinical benefit is not fully established, the proper evaluation does provide the framework for establishing the benefit of various hematopoietic growth factors now available for use.

PERIPHERAL BLOOD STEM CELL TRANSPLANTATION

The enrichment of circulating hematopoietic progenitor cells during the administration of G-CSF and GM-CSF has been exploited clinically by using either primed PBSC alone or for supplementing marrow. Peripheral blood stem cells that were collected during the administration of GM-CSF in the rebound phase of leukocyte recovery, especially after cyclophosphamide therapy, and that were then reinfused at the time of marrow reinfusion accelerates the recovery of neutrophils and platelets. Further modifications of the dose of growth factor and addition of new factors like IL-3, stem cell factor, PIXY 321 may further improve the quality of hematopoietic engraftment.[8,9,28,29] It has recently been reported that increased levels of hematopoietic growth factors are observed de novo in the serum of patients receiving chemotherapy with or without BMT. The levels are usually lower than those which are noted in patients on growth factors. This balance, especially with other interleukins, needs further evaluation.[30-33]

The role of erythropoietin alone or in combination with other hematopoietic growth factors in treatment of high dose cytotoxic therapy with transplantation needs to be further developed. It appears that erythropoietin may have clinical benefit in improving anemia especially when it is caused by drugs which are toxic to the kidney, i.e., cisplatinum.[34-36]

Better planning of post-transplant medications, especially hematopoietic growth factors, can significantly improve engraftment and may one day offer hope of out-patient management of patients undergoing intermediate- or high-dose chemotherapy.

REFERENCES

1. Jones RJ, Sharkis SJ, Celano P, Colvin OM, Rowley SC, Sensenbrenner LL: Progenitor cell assays predict hematopoietic reconstitution after syngeneic transplantation in mice. Blood 1987; 70:1186-1192.
2. Gulati SC, Yahalom J, Portlock C: Autologous bone transplantation In: Current problems in cancer. Haskell C, Canellos G, Portlock (eds). Mosby Year Book Publishers, NY 1991; 15:1-57.
3. Douay L, Gorin NC, Mary J-Y, Lemarie E, Lopez M, Najman A, Stachowiak J, Giarratana M-C, Bailou C, Salmon C, Duhamel G: Recovery of CFU-GM from cryopreserved bone marrow and in vivo evaluation after autologous bone marrow transplantation are predictive of engraftment. Exp Hematol 1986; 14:358-365.
4. Fritsch G, Emminger W, Buchinger P, Printz D, Gadner H: CD-34+ cell proportions in peripheral blood correlate with colony-forming capacity. Exp Hematol 1991; 19:1079-1083.
5. Siena S, Bregni M, Brando B, Belli N, Ravagnani F, Gandola L, Stern AC, Landsdorp PM, Bonadonna G, Ganni AM: Flow cytometry for clinical estimation of circulating hematopoietic progenitors for autologous transplantation in cancer patients. Blood 1991; 77:400-409.

6. Janssen WE, Farmelo MJ, Lee C, Smilee R, Kronish L, Elfenbein GJ: The CD34+ cell fraction in bone marrow and blood is not universally predictive of CFU-GM. Exp Hematol 1992; 20:528-530.

7. Siena S, Bregni M, Gianni AM, Janssen WE: Estimation of peripheral blood CD34+ cells for autologous transplantation in cancer patients: Exp Hematol 1993; 21:203-205.

8. Lieschke GJ, Burgess AW: Granulocyte colony-stimulating factor and granulocyte-macrophage colony-stimulating factor. N Eng J Med 1992; 327:28-35.

9. Lieschke GJ, Burgess AW: Granulocyte colony-stimulating factor and granulocyte-macrophage colony-stimulating factor. N Eng J Med 1992; 327:99-106.

10. DeWitte T, Gratwohl A, Van Der Lely N, Bacigalupo A, Stern AC, Speck B, Schattenberg A, Nissen C, Gluckman E, Fibbe WE: Recombinant human granulocyte-macrophage colony-stimulating factor accelerates neutrophil and monocyte recovery after allogeneic T-cell-depleted bone marrow transplantation. Blood 1992; 79:1359-1365.

11. Atkinson K, Biggs JC, Downs K, Juttner C, Bradstock K, Lowenthal RM, Dale B, Szer J: GM-CSF after allogeneic bone marrow transplantation: accelerated recovery of neutrophils, monocytes and lymphocytes. Aust NZ J Med 1991; 21:686-692.

12. Nemunaitis J, Rabinowe SN, Singer JW, Bierman PJ, Vose JM, Freedman AS, Onetto N, Gillis S, Oette D, Gold M, Buckner D, Hansen JA, Ritz J, Appelbaum FR, Armitage JO, Nadler LM: Recombinant granulocyte-macrophage colony-stimulating factor after autologous bone marrow transplantation for lymphoid cancer. N Eng J Med 1991; 324:1773-1778.

13. Gianni AM, Bregni M, Stern AC, Siena S, Tarella C, Pileri A, Bonadonna G: Granulocyte-macrophage colony-stimulating factor to harvest circulating haemopoietic stem cells for autotransplantation. Lancet 1989; 580-585.

14. Gulati SC, Bennett CL: Granulocyte-macrophage colony-stimulating factor (GM-CSF) as adjunct therapy in relapsed Hodgkin Disease. Annals of Internal Medicine 1992; 116:177-182.

15. Bot FJ, van Eijk L, Schipper P, Backx B, Lowenberg B: Synergistic effects between GM-CSF and G-CSF or M-CSF on highly enriched human marrow progenitor cells. Leukemia 1990; 4:325-328.

16. Morstyn G, Campbell L, Lieschke G, Layton JE, Maher D, O'Connor M, Green M, Sheridan W, Vincent M, Alton K, Souza L, McGrath K, Fox RM: Treatment of chemotherapy-induced neutropenia by subcutaneously administered granulocyte colony-stimulating factor with optimization of dose and duration of therapy. J Clin Oncol 1989; 7:1554-1562.

17. Bender JG, Bik To L, Williams S, Schwartzberg LS: Defining a therapeutic dose of peripheral blood stem cells. J of Hematotherapy 1992; 1:329-341.

18. To LB, Haylock DN, Dyson PG, Thorp D, Roberts MM, Juttner CA: An unusual patter of hematopoietic reconstitution in patients with acute myeloid leukemia transplanted with autologous recovery phase peripheral blood. Bone Marrow Transplant 1990; 5:109-114.

19. Harrison DE, Jordan CT, Zhong RK, Astle CM: Primitive hemopoietic stem cells: direct assay of most productive populations by competitive repopulation with simple binomial, correlation and covariance calculations. Exp Hematol 1993; 21:206-219.

20. Lopez M, Mary J-Y, Sainteny F: In vitro purging of bone marrow with mafosfamide synergizes with in vivo chemotherapy to delay the hematological recovery in a murine model of autologous bone marrow transplantation. Exp Hematol 1993; 21:311-318.

21. MacKintosh FR, Adlish J, Hall SW, St.Joer S, Smith E, Tavassoli M, Zanjani ED: Suppression of normal human hematopoiesis by cytomegalovirus in vitro. Exp Hematol 1993 21:243-250.

22. Childs B, Emanuel D: Cytomegalovirus infection and compromise. Exp Hematol 1993; 21:198-200.

23. Schwartzberg LS, Birch R, Hazelton B, Tauer KW, Lee P Jr, Altemose R, George C, Blanco R, Wittlin F, Cohen J, Muscato J, West WH: Peripheral blood stem cell mobilization by chemotherapy with or without recombinant human granulocyte colony-stimulating factor. J Hematotherapy 1992; 1:317-327.

24. Fleischhauer K, Kernan N, O'Reilly RJ, Dupont B, Young Yang S: Bone marrow-allograft rejection by T-lymphocytes recognizing a single amino acid difference in HLA-B44. N Engl J Med 1990; 323:1381-1822.

25. Emerson SG, Sieff CA, Gross RG, Rozans MK, Miller RA, Rappeport JM, Nathan DG: Decreased hematopoietic accessory cell function following bone marrow transplantation. Exp Hematol 1987; 15:1013-1021.

26. Straus SE, Cohen JI, Tosato G, Meier J: Epstein-Barr virus infections: Biology, pathogenesis, and management. Annals of Internal Medicine 1993; 118:45-58.

27. Anderson LJ, Torok T: Human Parvovirus B19. NEJM 1989; 321:536-538.

28. Neidhart J, Mangalik A, Stidley C, Tebich S, Sarmiento L, Pfile J, Oette D, Oldhan F: Dosing regimen of granulocyte-macrophage colony-stimulating factor to support dose-intensive chemotherapy. J Clin Oncol 1992; 10:1460-1469.

29. Jakubowski A, Raptis G, Gilewski T, Gabrilove J, Schuster S, Crown J, Hudis C, Seidman A, Hoffman R, Caron D: A phase I/II trial of PIXY 321 in patients with metastatic breast cancer receiving doxorubicin and thiotepa. Blood 1992; 80(Suppl 1):342.

30. Wing EJ, Magee DM, Whiteside TL, Kaplan SS, Shadduck RK: Recombinant human granulocyte-macrophage colony-stimulating factor enhances monocyte cytotoxicity and secretion of tumor necrosis factor α and interferon in cancer patients. Blood 1989; 73:643-646.

31. Haas R, Gericke G, Witt B, Cayeux S, Hunstein W: Increased serum levels of granulocyte colony-stimulating factor after autologous bone marrow or blood stem cell transplantation. Exp Hematol 1993; 21:109-113.

32. Kawano Y, Takaue Y, Saito S-I, Sato J, Shimuzu T, Suzue T, Hirao A, Okamoto Y, Abe T, Watanabe T, Kuroda Y, Kimura F, Motoyoshi K, Asano S: Granulocyte colony-stimulating factor macrophage-CSF, granulocyte-macrophage CSF, interleukin-3, and interleukin-6 levels in sera

from children undergoing blood stem cell autografts. Blood 1993; 81:856-860.

33. Barry MA, Behnke CA, Eastman A: Activation of programmed cell death (apoptosis) by cisplatin, other anticancer drugs, toxins and hyperthermia. Biochemical Pharmacology 1990; 40:2353-2362.

34. Locatelli F, Pedrazzoli P, Barosi G, Zecca M, Porta F, Liberato L, Gambarana D, Nespoli L, Cassola M: Recombinant human erythropoietin is effective in correcting erythropoietin-deficient anemia after allogeneic bone marrow transplantation. British J Haematol 1992; 80:545-549.

35. Miller CB, Platanias LC, Mills SR, Zahurak ML, Ratain MJ, Ettinger DS, Jones RJ: Phase I-II trial of erythropoietin in the treatment of cisplatin-associated anemia. J Natl Cancer Inst 1992; 84:98-103.

36. Platanias LC, Miller CB, Mick R, Hart RD, Ozer H, McEvilly J-M, Jones RJ, Ratain MJ: Treatment of chemotherapy-induced anemia with recombinant human erythropoietin in cancer patients. J Clin Oncol 1991; 9:2021-2026.

CHAPTER 8

FUTURE DIRECTIONS

Cancer cells are difficult to diagnose once the total-body burden is below 1 gram, which represents approximately one billion cells (Chapter 1, Figure 1). As discussed in Chapter 1, the number of cancer cells harvested during hematopoietic stem cell (HSC) removal when the patient is in apparent remission is usually unknown and most likely effects the subsequent outcome of autologous stem cell transplantation (AUSCT). How the human body clears the minimal cancer burden is not fully known. The disease reoccurs from minimal residual disease (MRD), and further work is needed to study minimal tumor burden.

DRUG RESISTANCE

Often the recurring cells after purged stem cell transplant (SCT) demonstrate drug resistance.[1-6] We must understand the various biological changes and drug resistance mechanisms of each "cancer-treatment combination." Considering that drug resistance starts to develop with the first exposure to cytotoxic drugs, one approach could be to try to decrease drug resistance by early institution of drugs which decrease the development of drug resistance, e.g., verapamil and cyclosporine. Newer analogues of cyclosporine and verapamil (bepridil) are now under clinical investigations to avoid the clinical toxicity of the two drugs.[3,4] These maneuvers may decrease the drug-resistant cells and improve the success of subsequent stem cell harvesting and thus transplantation.[3,4]

In one study, a combined approach for purging multidrug resistant leukemic cell lines in bone marrow using a monoclonal antibody [17F9, directed against the cell surface product of the multiple drug resistance (MDR) gene, P-glycoprotein] and chemotherapy was attempted. Using two different cell lines, the investigators demonstrated that 17F9+ complement (C') selectively lyses MDR-positive cells. Three rounds of antibody + C' resulted in 96.4% ± 3.6% kill of K562/DOX (a human erythroleukemia cell line resistant to doxorubicin) and 100% ± 0% of CEM/VLB (a human lymphoblastic leukemia cell line selected to be resistant to velban) cells. Mixtures of malignant cells and normal BM resulted in 99.85% removal of K562/DOX and 99.91% removal of CEM/VLB clonogenic cells. This treatment did not affect normal committed precursors compared with C' alone. The addition of the cytotoxic agent etoposide (VP-16) following antibody purging results in a 4.6 log reduction of malignant cells. Furthermore, this antibody was effective when used against patients' leukemic blasts. These results suggest that the use of 17F9 + C' is effective and selective for removal of MDR cells from BM before ABMT and the addition of VP-16 enhances the purging efficacy.[5]

We have evaluated the potential role of photoradiation therapy with a benzoporphyrin derivative, monoacid ring A (BPD-MA), and dihemato-porphyrin ether (DHE), for the ex vivo purging of residual tumor cells, especially with the intent to see if these compounds will be useful once drug resistance has developed.[6] BPD-MA and DHE photosensitizing activity was tested against two human large-cell lymphoma cell lines and colony-forming unit-leukemia (CFU-L) derived from patients with acute myelogenous leukemia (AML). In mixing experiments, 4-log elimination of tumor cell lines was observed after 1 hour of incubation with 75 ng/mL of BPD-MA or 30 minutes of treatment with 12.5 g/mL of DHE followed by white light exposure. By comparison, using the same concentration of BPD-MA, the mean recovery of normal BM progenitors was 4% ± 0.8% (mean ± SD) for granulocyte-macrophage colony-forming unit (CFU-GM) and 5% ± 0.8% for burst-forming unit-erythroid (BFU-e). Similarly, DHE treatment resulted in the recovery of 5.2% ± 2% and 9.8% ± 3% of CFU-GM and BFU-e, respectively. Furthermore, equivalently cytotoxic concentrations of both DHE and BPD-MA and light were found not to kill normal pluripotent stem cells in BM. This was demonstrated by similar survival of the treated cells to the controls in "two-step long-term marrow culture". The T-lymphoblastic leukemia cell line CEM and its vinblastine (VBL)-resistant subline CEM/VBL, along with the acute promyelocyte leukemia cell line HL-60 and its vincristine (VCR)-resistant subline HL-60/VCR, were also tested. BPD-MA at 75 ng/mL was able to provide a greater than 4-log elimination of the drug-sensitive cell lines, but only a 34% and 55% decrease of the drug-resistant HL-60/VCR and CEM/VBL cell lines, respectively. In contrast, 12.5 mcg/mL of DHE reduced the clonogenic growth of all the cell lines by more than 4 logs. Further experiments demonstrated decreased uptake of BPD-MA and DHE by the resistant cell lines. However, all the cell lines took up more DHE than BPD-MA under similar experimental conditions. Normal early hematopoietic cells can express MDR[7] and this observation should be considered in purging methods, the investigators did not find this to be a significant problem.[6] These results demonstrate the preferential cytotoxicity of BPD-MA and DHE toward neoplastic cell lines and CFU-L from AML patients. In addition, DHE was slightly more effective in purging tumor cells expressing the p-170 glycoprotein. Recent data suggests that alkyl-lysophospholids (ALP) may also retain cytotoxicity towards conventional drug-resistant malignant cells.[8] These results suggest that newer approaches could be developed and incorporated into clinical trials with the intent of decreasing residual drug-resistant leukemia and lymphoma.[6,9]

ONCOGENES

Viral involvement in pathophysiology of lymphoma and Hodgkin's disease and its contribution to the alteration of biological behavior and thus "treatment planning" needs further investigations.[12-15] Post-transplant (BMT, renal and heart) lymphomas show abnormal expression of EBV, and often respond to biological response modifiers. In one recent study, expression of Epstein-Barr virus encoded small RNA (EBER-1 gene product) was noted in post-transplantation lymphoproliferative disorders (PTLD) and EBER-1 gene expression in liver tissue precedes the occurrence of clinical and histologic PTLD. This observation may provide tools for early diagnosis of lymphoma. Early intervention in appropriately selected patients may decrease the problems related to the emergence of drug resistance, bulky disease, etc. The role of tumor suppressor genes (p53, etc.) and other oncogenes in initial causation and possible progression of malignancy needs to be better understood as it is possible that such patients with suppressor gene alteration will respond to different purging strategy.[12,13] Proper understanding of these mechanisms will facilitate the patient's in vivo and ex vivo treatment. In one recent report, a T-cell acute lymphoblastic leukemia (T-ALL) cell line was found to have alteration in p53 and the defect was correctable by the insertion of wild type p53 gene.[13] Similarly, clones of CML can be inhibited by antisense genes.[14]

HEMATOPOIETIC GROWTH FACTORS

The increasing use of hematopoietic growth factor with BMT was discussed in Chapter 7 and has decreased the duration of neutropenia. Several recent trials have occasionally utilized hematopoietic growth factor rescue after partial hematoablation. Even though the long-term toxicity and side effects of hematopoietic growth factors are not well known, use of GM-CSF, G-CSF (without hematopoietic stem cell rescue) is probably safer than the risks of hematopoietic stem cell transplantation. For each drug we need to know more about how much "dose-escalation" is possible before the need for stem cell transplantation (Chapter 1, Figure 2). The figure also describes this window (higher drug dose with growth factor but without SCT) which needs to be further explored. We also need to investigate new growth factors and evaluate different combinations as we still need improvements in the speed of engraftment of erythroid and megakaryocytic series. Furthermore, we still need to know more about the therapeutic benefit of multiple cycles of higher dose therapy given over a short period of time (without transplant) when compared to one (or two) cycle of hematoablative dosage with hematopoietic stem cell rescue. These highly aggressive therapies need to be better designed to keep therapeutic and economic benefits in perspective.[16-21] The growth factors can also be utilized to expand hematopoietic cells in tissue culture. This approach may prove to have a significant purging advantage, as special culture media can be developed which allow the preferential growth of presumed normal hematopoietic cells over the malignant cells.[21,22] Furthermore, factors which protect normal tissue during purging can be used more efficiently.[22-25] Collection of PBSCs is also a reasonable alternative for patients whose bone marrow is technically difficult to aspirate or for patients with previous radiation to the sites of BM harvest.

STEM CELL ENRICHMENT

The human CD-34 hematopoietic stem cell antigen is a highly glycosylated type 1 membrane protein of unknown function. CD-34 is expressed on 1% to 4% of bone marrow cells, including pluripotent stem cells and committed progenitors of each hematopoietic lineage. CD-34 has also been shown to be expressed on the small vessel endothelium of a variety of tissues and on a subset of bone marrow stromal cells.[26] Understanding the regulatory mechanisms involved in CD-34 expression will help in designing better methods for enriching CD-34 cells. Recently, it was shown that the CD-34 gene is transcriptionally regulated in tissue culture cells. Further understanding of this CD-34 promoter should result in the identification of stem cell/progenitor cell-specific transcription factors and should provide a means to direct the expression of heterologous genes in hematopoietic stem cells and progenitors. The growth can be further augmented by the use of growth factors and special microenvironment systems available.[20,21,27-31]

RESOURCES USED AND COST

Significant concern now exists about the escalating medical costs. Often the cost varies from one institution to another, and cost to the provider is different than the cost to the consumer. One approach is to evaluate the resources used. For example, bone marrow harvest (BMH), which can now be done in the out-patient operating room, and PBSCT transplant, which is also useful for autologous SCT, have different amount of resources used. In this regard, the comparison should be made of the: 1) resources used: i.e., time spent by patient (loss of productivity if patient is employed), doctors, nurses, laboratory technicians, secretaries, etc. and money spent on supplies; 2) cost to the hospital; 3) cost to the patient; and 4) decrease in cost of subsequent high dose therapy with SCT rescue.[16]

ALLOGENEIC BMT

For patients undergoing allogeneic BMT, better management of graft-versus-host disease and graft rejection will significantly help improve the disease free survival of the patients. Approaches which need further evaluation include selective depletion of lymphocytes from the bone marrow (CD-5, CD-8, etc. depletion, partial T-cell removal) and improvements in post-transplant management of graft-versus-host disease, and relapse. Exploiting the advantage of graft-versus-cancer is another significant approach.[32] Infusion of donor lymphocytes, causing transient GVHD, immunopotentiation (especially post-transplant) etc. are some of the new exciting possibilities.[33-35] Use of alternate sources of stem cells (umbilical blood, cadaveric marrow, national unrelated donor registries) needs further exploration, perhaps with methods of stem cell expansion.[21,36] (See also Chapters 1,2 and 4.)

GENE THERAPY

Newer methods of gene transfer may allow preferential in vitro growth of normal hematopoietic precursors with increased drug tolerance and an increased immunosurveillance armatorium. Expression of the human multiple drug resistance (MDR) gene confers resistance to a variety of compounds in vitro and in vivo. In order to determine the feasibility of conferring recipient erythroid cells drug resistance for the MDR phenotype, investigators have transduced mouse erythroleukemia cells (MELC) with the MDR gene in a retroviral vector. MELC clones resistant to colchicine (an MDR-responsive agent) can be isolated, and demonstrate high levels of MDR RNA and protein expression. Increasing doses of colchicine increase the level of MDR RNA and protein expression significantly. These results indicate that it is possible to transfer and express the human MDR phenotype in mouse erythroid cells by retrovirally mediated gene transfer, and that drug selection can be used to enrich or purify populations of cells containing and expressing this gene. Other approaches to explore these findings and clinical protocols utilizing the concerns of drug resistance need to be developed.[9]

As mentioned in Chapter 1, bone marrow harvested for autologous bone marrow transplantation may contain residual malignant cells, even after appropriate purging and clinically these patients are usually judged to be in remission. Genetic marking of the purged cells infused at SCT and subsequent detection in the recipients would give useful information about the origin of relapse after transplantation. In one recent study, neomycin-resistance gene was transferred into bone-marrow cells harvested from children with acute myeloid leukemia in remission. Two patients relapsed after reinfusion of the marked cells. In both, the resurgent blast cells contained the neomycin-resistance gene marker; thus, remission marrow can contribute to disease recurrence. This method of tracking malignant cells should enable the evaluation marrow purging strategies.[37,38]

POST-TRANSPLANT TREATMENT

There is now a significant interest in post-transplant immunomodulatory therapy to decrease the relapse from the possible small number of cancer cells still present after conditioning regimen and/or from concomitant infusion of cancer cells with transplantation. Immunotoxin tagged antibodies against cancer cells are now being evaluated for post-transplant erradication of minimal disease.[39] Immunopotentiator drugs (Linomide, IL-2) are also under clinical investigation.[40-42] Linomide stimulates natural killer cells, T-cells and monocytes in patients with AML who underwent autologous BMT.[41] It has already shown promising results in controlling autoimmune disease in rodents. International double blind (placebo vs. linomide) trial is ongoing for postautologous stem cell transplant treatment of patients with acute myeloblastic leukemia.

THE PURPOSE OF LIFE IS A LIFE OF PURPOSE. —ROBERT BYRNE

The use (purpose) of high-dose chemotherapy, purging and stem cell transplantation has shown the most benefit for patients with acute myeloblastic leukemia and lymphoma. It is often hard to discern if the success is due to patient selection, high-dose chemotherapy or purging conditions. The advantage may even be in treatment planning and may depend on both the conditioning regimen and purging method. (See Chapter 6, Table 3.) Treatment plans for diseases with approximately 50-60% long-term disease-free survival (LT-DFS) cause a dilemma for the design of future trials. For example: Should we continue to perform phase I/II studies until we attain 70-90% success? Or should we prove the therapeutic benefit of the transplant protocol in phase III randomized trial against the best possible conventional therapy, or prove the need of purging in a randomized, preferably double blind trial? Placing too much emphasis on proving (if possible) clinical benefit of strategies with 50-60% LT-DFS will deter development of protocols with the possibility of 70-90% success.

Randomized clinical trials for disease with less than 40% LT-DFS are even harder to justify and these trials can focus on first improving and proving the clinical benefit of the treatment before concentrating on deciding the best form of hematopoietic support or cost analysis. Unfortunately, clinical trials often get involved in proving the tolerability of expensive transplant schedules with moderate changes in "drug(s)-dose schedules" and do not address the question of clinical benefit. Furthermore, the success of hematopoietic rescue will change with alterations in re-induction and/or higher dosages of transplant conditioning regimen; thus the analysis of "speed of engraftment" of various hematopoietic lineages will have to be reevaluated and considered in the wider context of long-term benefits. Does inadvertent infusion of cancer cells along with stem cell transplant (BM and/or PB) increase relapse rate (especially for disease known to have frequent bone marrow involvement)?

In other words: *How does 5-10 days benefit in "speed of hematopoietic engraftment" or decrease in the "days of hospitalization" balance against "increased possibility of relapse"?* A subtle increase in the relapse rate has not been properly evaluated in the published clinical trials.

From the details provided in this book, one can summarize that significant progress has been made in developing the purging methods for bone marrow transplantation. The complexity of issues and our inability to properly quantitate minimal disease for most cancers has weakened the scientific justification for purging. Future trials should focus on proving the benefit of each significant variable. Overall, the success of purged stem cell transplantation has improved, and a good portion of the patients can now enjoy a better quality of life.

REFERENCES

1. Niehans GA, Waclaw J, Brunetto V: Immunohistochemical identification of P-glycoprotein in previously untreated diffuse large cell and immunoblastic lymphomas. Cancer Res 1992; 52:3768-3775.

2. Verrelle P, Meissonier F, Fonck Y: Clinical relevance of immunohistochemical detection of multidrug resistance of P-glycoprotein in breast carcinoma. JNCI 1991 83:111-116.

3. van Kalken CK, van der Hoeven JJM, der Jong J: Bepridil in combination with anthracyclines to reverse anthracycline resistance in cancer patients. Eur J Cancer 1991; 27:739-744.

4. Sonneveld P, Durie BGM, Lokhorst HM: Modulation of multidrug-resistant multiple myeloma by cyclosporin. Lancet 1992; 340:255-259.

5. Aihara M, Aihara Y, Schmidt-Wolf G, Schmidt-Wolf I, Sikic BI, Blume KG, Chao NJ: A combined approach for purging multidrug-resistant leukemic cell lines in bone marrow using a monoclonal antibody and chemotherapy. Blood 1991; 77:2079-2084.

6. Lemoli RM, Igarashi T, Knizewski M, Acaba L, Richter A, Jain A, Mitchell D, Levy J, Gulati SC: Dye-mediated photolysis is capable of eliminating drug-resistant MDR tumor cells. Blood 1993; 81:793-800.

7. Chaudhary PM, Roninson IB: Expression and activity of P-glycoprotein, a multidrug efflux pump, in human hematopoietic cells. Cell 1991; 66:85-94.

8. Glasser L, Fiederlein RL, Dalton WS, Vogler WR: The effect of alkyl-lysophospholipids on human myeloma cell lines. Blood 1992; 80(Suppl 1):484.

9. DelaFlor-Weiss E, Richardson C, Ward M, Himelstein A, Smith L, Podda S, Gottesman M, Pastan I, Bank A: Transfer and expression of the human multidrug resistance gene in mouse erythroleukemia cells. Blood 1992; 80:3106-3111.

10. Cesarman E, Chadburn A, Inghirami G, Gaidano G, Knowles DM:

Structural and functional analysis of oncogenes and tumor suppressor genes in adult T-cell leukemia/lymphoma shows frequent p53 mutations. Blood 1992; 80:3205-3216.

11. Randhawa PS, Jaffe R, Demetris AJ, Nalesnik M, Starzl TE, Chen YY, Weiss LM: Expression of Epstein-Barr virus-encoded small RNA (by the eber-1 gene) in liver specimens from transplant recipients with posttransplantation lymphoproliferative disease. N Engl J Med 1992; 327:1710-1714.

12. Vaux DL, Weissman IL, Kim SK: Prevention of programmed cell death in caenorhabditis elegan by human bcl-2. Science 1992; 258:1955-1958.

13. Cheng J, Yee J-K, Yeargin J, Friedmann T, Haas M: Suppression of acute lymphoblastic leukemia by the human wild-type p53 gene. Cancer Research 1992; 52:222-226.

14. Martiat P, Lewalle P, Taj AS, Philippe M, Larondelle Y, Vaerman JL, Wilsmann C, Goldman JM, Michaux JL: Retrovirally transduced antisense sequences stably suppress P210 bcr-abl expression and inhibit the proliferation of bcr/abl-containing cell lines. Blood 1993; 81:502-509.

15. Pagano JS: Epstein-Barr virus: Culprit or consort? NEJM 1992; 327:1750-1752.

16. Gulati SC, Bennett C, Phillips J, Van-Poznak C: GM-CSF as an adjunct to autologous bone marrow transplantation. Stem Cells 1993; 11:20-25.

17. Crown J, Kritz A, Vahdat L, Reich L, Hamilton N, Harrison M, D;Aluta R, Fennelly D, Schneider J, Gilewski T, Hudis C, Motzer R, Connors C, Moore M, Gulati SC, Norton L: Feasibility of multiple, rapidly cycled courses of high-dose chemotherapy, supported by G-CSF and peripheral blood progenitors in patients with metastatic breast cancer. Blood 1992; 80(Supp 1):2074.

18. Siena S, Bregni M, Gianni AM, Janssen WE: Estimation of peripheral blood CD34+ cells for autologous transplantation in cancer patients. Exp Hematol 1993; 21:203-205.

19. Lieschke GJ, Burgess AW: Granulocyte colony-stimulating factor and granu-locyte-macrophage colony-stimulating factor. N Eng J Med 1992; 327:28-35.

20. Lieschke GJ, Burgess AW: Granulocyte colony-stimulating factor and granu-locyte-macrophage colony-stimulating factor. N Eng J Med 1992; 327:99-106.

21. Lemoli RM, Tafuri A, Strife A, Andreeff M, Clarkson BD, Gulati SC: Proliferation of human hematopoietic progenitors in long-term bone marrow cultures in gas-permeable plastic bags is enhanced by colony-stimulating factors. Exp Hematol 1992; 20:569-575.

22. Moore MAS: Does stem cell exhaustion result from combining hemato-poietic growth factors with chemotherapy? If so, how do we prevent it? Blood 1992; 80:3-7.

23. Lemoli RM, Strife A, Clarkson BD, Haley JD, Gulati SC: TGF-beta 3 protects normal human hematopoietic progenitor cells treated with 4-HC in vitro. Exp Hematol 1992; 20:1252-1256.

24. Stemmer SM, Shpall EJ, Jones RB, Hami L, Bearman SI, Myers SE, Taffs S, Shaw L, Capizzi RL, Schein P: Amifostine (WR-2721) shortens the engraftment time of 4-HC purged bone marrow in lymphoma patients receiving high-dose chemotherapy with autologous bone marrow sup-

port. Blood 1992; 80(Suppl 1):269.

25. Bonewald LF: Can transforming growth factor beta be useful as a protective agent for pluripotent hematopoietic progenitor cells? Exp Hematol 1992; 20:1249-1251.

26. Burn TC, Satterthwaite AB, Tenen DG: The human CD-34 hematopoietic stem cell antigen promoter and a 3' enhancer direct hematopoietic expression in tissue culture. Blood 1992; 80:3051-3059.

27. Gurevitch O, Fabian I: Ability of the hemopoietic microenvironment in the induced bone to maintain the proliferative potential of early hemopoietic precursors. Stem Cells 1993; 11:56-61.

28. McCarthy K, Weintroub S, Hale M, Reddi AH: Establishment of the hemopoietic microenvironment in the marrow of matrix-induced endochondral bone. Exp Hematol 1984; 12:131-138.

29. Brugger W, Frisch J, Schulz G, Pressler K, Mertelsmann R, Kanz L: Sequential administration of interleukin-3 and granulocyte-macrophage colony-stimulating factor following standard-dose combination chemotherapy with etoposide, ifosfamide, and cisplatin. J Clin Oncol 1992; 10:1452-1459.

30. Naparstek E, Hardan Y, Ben-Shahar M, Nagler A, Or R, Mumcuoglu M, Weiss L, Samuel S, Slavin S: Enhanced marrow recovery by short preincubation of marrow allografts with human recombinant interleukin-3 and granulocyte-macrophage colony-stimulating factor. Blood 1992; 80:1673-1678.

31. Pietsch T, Kyas U, Steffens U, Yakisan E, Hadam MR, Ludwig W-D, Zsebo K, Welte K: Effects of human stem cell factor (c-kit ligand) on proliferation of myeloid leukemia cells: Heterogeneity in response and synergy with other hematopoietic growth factors. Blood 1992; 80(Suppl 5):1199-1206.

32. Hess AD, Jones RJ, Morris LE, Noga SJ, Vogelsang GB, Santos GW: Autologous graft-versus-host disease: A novel approach for antitumor immunotherapy. Hum Immunol 1992; 34:219-224.

33. Nierle T, Bunjes D, Arnold R, Heimpel H, Theobald M: Quantitative assessment of post-transplant host-specific interleukin-2-secreting T-helper cell precursors in patients with and without acute graft-versus-host disease after allogeneic HLA-identical sibling bone marrow transplantation. Blood 1993; 81:841-848.

34. Blazar BR, Widmer MB, Taylor PA, Vallera DA: Promotion of murine marrow alloengraftment and hematopoietic recovery across the major histocompatibility barrier by administration of recombinant human interleukin-α. Blood 1992; 80:1614-1622.

35. Schwarer AP, Jiang YZ, Brookes PA, Barret AJ, Batchelor JR, Goldman JM, Lechler RI: Frequency of anti-recipient alloreactive helper T-cell precursors in donor blood and graft-versus-host disease after HLA-identical sibling bone marrow transplantation. Lancet 1993; 341:203-204.

36. Broxmeyer HE, Hangoc G, Cooper S, Ribeiro RC, Graves V, Yoder M, Wagner J, Vadhan-Raj S, Benninger L, Rubinstein P, Broun ER: Growth characteristics and expansion of human umbilical cord blood and estimation of its potential for transplantation in adults. Proc Natl Acad Sci 1992; 89:4109-4113.

37. Brenner MK, Rill DR, Moen RC, Krance RA, Mirro J Jr, Anderson WF, Ihle JN: Gene-marking to trace origin of relapse after autologous bone-marrow transplantation. Lancet 1993; 341:85-86.

38. Gross S: To purge or not to purge is not the question. J of Hematotherapy 1992; 1:299-301.

39. Grossbard ML, Freedman AS, Ritz J, Coral F, Goldmacher VS, Eliseo L, Spector N, Dear K, Lambert JM, Battler WA, Taylor JM, Nadler LM: Serotherapy of B-cell neoplasms with anti-B4-blocked ricin: A phase I trial of daily bolus infusion. Blood 1992; 79:576-585.

40. Gerdin B, Wanders A, Tufveson G: Rat cardiac allografts protected with cyclosporin A are rejected in the presence of LS-2616 (Linomide). Transplantation Proceedings 1989; 21:853-855.

41. Bengtsson M, Simonsson B, Carlsson K, Nilsson BI, Smedmyr B, Termander B, Oberg G, Totterman TH: Stimulation of NK cell, T cell, and monocyte functions by the novel immunomodulator linomide after autologous bone marrow transplantation. Transplantation 1992; 53:882-888.

42. Simonsson B, Nilsson BI, Rowe JM: Treatment of minimal residual disease in acute leukemia - focus on immunotherapeutic options. Leukemia 1992; 6(Suppl 4):124-134.

INDEX